TAKE BACK YOUR LIFE

Find Hope And Freedom From
Fibromyalgia Symptoms And Pain

Tami Stackelhouse

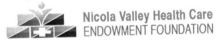

ISBN: 978-1-942646-58-7

Cover Design & Page Design: John H. Matthews

Editing: Kate Makled

Author's photo courtesy of Rayleigh Leavitt. Photography by Rayleigh

SPECIAL DISCLAIMER:

*For you
and all the women with fibromyalgia
who have felt like prisoners in their own
bodies.*

There is hope. You can be free.

ADVANCE PRAISE

In *Take Back Your Life*, Tami takes an honest look at fibromyalgia and expertly discusses long-term management since there is no cure. She teaches the value of self-care and an integrative, multi-faceted approach to live a better quality of life. Her writing breaks down the challenges that keep us stuck in not knowing what to do next by offering new ideas and approaches.

Jan Favero Chambers, President
National Fibromyalgia & Chronic Pain
Association
FMcpAware.org

With an inviting blend of honesty and optimism, *Take Back Your Life* provides a path toward healing and understanding for those living with fibromyalgia. Stackelhouse delivers scientific and anecdotal knowledge in a seasoned voice born from her personal journey and passion for helping others.

Dr. Kaley Bourgeois
Lake Oswego Health Center, PC
LakeOswegoHealth.com

I highly recommend *Take Back Your Life* as a go-to resource for current information, tips, and resources to get started or as a reference for any part of your fibromyalgia wellness journey. You will love Tami's rubber–meets-the-road approach, as she shares her own experiences combined with scientific knowledge and possibilities for making a successful difference in your own life.

Cindy Sharp, VP of Leadership Development
National Fibromyalgia & Chronic Pain
Association, FMcpAware.org

It is so wonderful that Tami has taken the time to create this resource for those dealing with fibromyalgia. When I was diagnosed as a teenager it was a crazy maze of doctors and alternative treatments and trying to convince my family and friends that there was actually something wrong with me because I didn't look sick. To know that a resource like this exists brings happy tears of gratitude to my eyes!

Megan Densmore
Chronic Illness Advocate, Actor, Athlete
Invisible-Film.com

Take Back Your Life is truly a valuable guidebook for anyone living with fibromyalgia.

Tami has provided a wealth of information to aid in understanding this complex health challenge in a very succinct and easy to read format. In addition, she offers an abundance of concrete and practical suggestions to help you shortcut the trying frustrations of trial and error. Tami's coaching style shines thru on every page.

Elaine Merryfield
Adult health / wellness educator
Specializing in both fibromyalgia and stress relief
NavigatingLifeWithFibro.com

Tami Stackelhouse is ahead of her time in her approach to working with Fibromyalgia. Her own experience with this malady gives an insiders perspective and offers a beacon of hope for those in need. Tami's holistic coaching empowers sufferers to manage this ailment in an effective way and to begin their journey toward healing.

Aram Levendosky
Licensed Acupuncturist
Acupuncture & Oriental Medicine-AOM Health
AOMHealth.com

I highly recommend *Take Back Your Life*. Having learned to manage her own fibromyalgia and being a Fibromyalgia Health Coach, Tami passes her experience and knowledge onto others so they do not have to spend their time researching what she has already done. If you have fibromyalgia and are looking for a book that is easy to read, offers helpful tips on living with fibromyalgia or want a better understanding on how to manage fibromyalgia symptoms this is the book for you.

Melissa Swanson
Chronic Pain Patient, Advocate, Author
Fibro Warriors – Living Life
SurvivingWithFibro.wordpress.com

In this book, Tami not only describes why fibromyalgia is like the elephant in the room, but also how to deal with this chronic beast of burden. She offers valid, productive treatment options in a way that is far from being a stiff medical read. The language and layout are easy, precise, and to the point, just like Ms. Stackelhouse's coaching sessions. If you want to take back your life from fibromyalgia, I highly recommend that you read *Take Back Your Life!*

Jenna Cooke, Editor
FibroDaily.com

TABLE OF CONTENTS

FOREWORD

Tami Stackelhouse is both a gifted health coach and a passionate advocate for people with fibromyalgia. I witnessed this firsthand when she and I testified together in front of the Oregon State Legislature to argue that fibromyalgia should be a covered diagnosis on the state Medicaid plan.

I had asked a patient who was unable to access healthcare due to this law, to give a statement about her experience. She was hesitant and worried that her brain was too foggy to speak clearly and effectively. Tami offered to call her the night before and help her prepare. When my patient walked up to the podium she told her story confidently and clearly, and I could see how much Tami's encouragement had helped her.

In *Take Back Your Life,* Tami provides the same type of encouragement to her readers. She includes useful guidance on how to pace activities to break the push/crash cycle and how to build your own health care team. Having the right providers on your team is vital to getting the help you need to feel better, and her advice on how to do this will be useful to every reader.

She gives great suggestions on things to try on your own to reduce symptoms, and is clear about which treatments to speak to a health care provider about first. She includes her own story, and that of some of her clients, so you can see how treatments work for real people in their lives.

She also gives powerful advice about caring and having compassion for yourself, or as she says "how to be on the same team as your body." Self-compassion can be challenging in an illness like fibromyalgia, when it's natural to feel frustrated and angry with your body. As someone with fibromyalgia, I know how hard this can be personally. Taking care of yourself, loving yourself—these are things I wish for all of my patients, and Tami beautifully describes how to do that in this book.

Ginevra Liptan, MD
Medical Director
The Frida Center for Fibromyalgia
Lake Oswego, Oregon

June 2015

INTRODUCTION

For most of my life, I've wondered what was wrong with me. I grew up with a steady diet of doctors and medical appointments. I never felt quite "normal." I was sick and tired often and had constant headaches.

The first time I thought I had found an answer for my fatigue and headaches was right after high school. I had read *The Low Blood Sugar Handbook* by Edward and Patricia Krimmel. Hypoglycemia (low blood sugar) explained a lot of my symptoms, but not all of them. I tried sticking to their suggestions for keeping blood sugar levels stable. It helped–a little. I still didn't feel "normal," whatever that was.

The next time I thought I'd found an answer was after reading *The Yeast Connection* by William G. Crook, M.D. I took his quiz to evaluate the likelihood that I was suffering from a candida overgrowth–and I scored off the charts! I called my parents. As soon as they answered the phone, I blurted out, "I know what's been wrong with me my whole life!" But I actually didn't. After trying dietary changes to reduce candida, and even some medical intervention, nothing about my health changed. I was still tired, still had headaches, and still wasn't "normal."

The next thing I started looking into was fibromyalgia and chronic fatigue syndrome. I bought Dr. Jacob Teitelbaum's book, *From Fatigued to Fantastic!* For the first time, everything seemed to fit: fatigue, brain fog, poor sleep, nagging body aches, and pain. It even explained why I always felt worse, and often got sick, after working out. It wasn't until I read his book that I realized how much pain I was actually in every day. I had thought that hurting in the evening was just a byproduct of living life. Never mind that I was in my mid-20s and had a desk job!

I sent my doctor an email explaining my symptoms and asked, "Is it possible that I have fibromyalgia or CFIDS?" (Chronic Fatigue Immune Dysfunction Syndrome, the name that was being used at that time.) Her medical assistant wrote back and said, "I'm not sure what that is. Why don't you make an appointment and we'll talk about it." Needless to say, I wasn't encouraged. At my appointment, I was told that I was probably just depressed due to working a very stressful job. I was referred to counseling. As you might imagine, counseling didn't do a whole lot for the pain or overwhelming fatigue I was experiencing. I gave up the idea that I would get help from my primary care physician and started trying to find it elsewhere.

I looked for anyone who was familiar with fibromyalgia, hypoglycemia, and candida overgrowth. I read anything I could get my hands on that might have an answer. I visited my first naturopath. The treatments he used definitely helped, but I had to pay for everything out of my own pocket; insurance wouldn't cover any of it. At 32 years old, and single, I couldn't keep paying hundreds of dollars a week for supplements, no matter how well they were working. I essentially gave up on finding an answer.

Three years later, I married my husband, Scott, and moved onto his insurance. This meant finding a new doctor. Scott and I looked online at possible doctors and picked one based on her photo and a short one-paragraph biography. We knew nothing else about her. On one hand, I was hopeful that she would give me answers. On the other hand, I wasn't expecting much because doctors had let me down for years. I spent several days before my first appointment writing down all of my symptoms, as well as my complicated medical history. I made notes on the medications I'd tried, what worked, and what hadn't. I basically armed myself for battle. I was going to get help, even if I had to fight for it.

After being with my doctor for just a few minutes, she said, "I think you have fibromyalgia." It turned out that treating fibromyalgia was one of her areas of expertise. I wanted to shout for joy! Someone was finally taking my symptoms seriously. I left her office with half a dozen new prescriptions, as well as a list of supplements to buy. I was in a daze. I didn't really want prescriptions, but I *did* want to feel better and was willing to try anything. I drove home in tears because someone *finally* believed that something was wrong. I was finally going to get help.

My doctor introduced me to a health coach two years into my fibromyalgia journey, and everything started to change. I learned how to take control of my own life and health. I decided that I wanted my pain and suffering to help others, so I became a coach. I started teaching other women with fibromyalgia what I had learned the hard way.

This book is a compilation of those things, written so that you can learn from my experiences. I want to save you the time and heartache I went through trying things that didn't work, in order to discover what did. Most of the things I discuss in this book are the things that your doctor can't do for you. They are the things that only you can do for yourself. Occasionally, I will discuss tests or medications that you can work on with your doctor. For the most part, however, this book contains the practical day-to-day, rubber-meets-the-road strategies that have helped me live a great life as a fibromyalgia patient.

HOW TO USE THIS BOOK

I've written this book so that it can be used two ways.

Option 1:
Read the book from front to back, in order.
The chapters are arranged in the order that I generally use with my coaching clients. These are the things that they struggle with most: pain, fatigue, poor sleep, and working with doctors. Please don't think that the latter chapters are somehow less important. They aren't. The last two chapters will help you to fine-tune what you've learned from the first chapters.

Choose this option if you:
- Are newly diagnosed with fibromyalgia.
- Haven't received effective fibromyalgia treatment, even if your diagnosis is not new.
- Want a refresher course on the basics before tackling more advanced topics.
- Love someone who has fibromyalgia and want to understand their illness and how you can help them better.

Option 2:
Choose your own adventure.
While all of the chapters in this book go together to treat the whole person, you can also skip around to the topics you need or want most. Your desire and enthusiasm, not to mention burning need, will take you a long way. Go with whatever jumps out at you first.

Choose this option if you:
- Have a particular symptom that is driving you crazy or severely limiting you in some way.
- Feel a burning desire to improve a particular area of your life.
- Feel stuck or overwhelmed. Sometimes it's okay to go with what feels easiest.
- Have most of your symptoms under control, but still have a few areas of your life you want to improve upon.
- Love someone with fibromyalgia, but have questions about specific symptoms or ways you can help.

Throughout this book, I'll be sharing bits of my own story and inviting you to connect with me. Please know that I mean every word of this. Helping other people, like you, gives meaning to the pain that I went through. Let my story be an example for you and a source of hope. I certainly haven't done everything perfectly. However, through trial, error, frustration, and heartache, I have found a way to thrive and live the life I want to live.

CHAPTER 1
WHAT DOES IT MEAN TO HAVE A FIBROMYALGIA DIAGNOSIS?

"The body speaks to us in whispers and when we ignore the whispers, the body starts to yell." – Lissa Rankin, MD

An old Indian parable tells of a group of blind men who try to figure out what an elephant looks like by touching it. Each man feels only one part of the elephant and describes the animal based on his experience. The man who feels the elephant's leg says, "An elephant is like a tree." The man who touches the tail says, "No. An elephant is like a rope." The one who puts his hands on the broad side of the elephant says, "I disagree. An elephant is like a wall." Another compares the elephant's ear to a hand fan, and so on. As they argue over which experience reveals the correct form of the elephant, a sighted man walks by. After receiving a description of the whole elephant, the blind men realize that each one's experience was simply a part of the whole.

I believe that fibromyalgia is like that elephant. Some scientists see the tail, while others see the leg or the ear. In 2013, there was a news article titled, "Fibromyalgia Mystery Finally Solved!"[1] The information in this article is good, but the title is misleading; it only describes one piece of the fibromyalgia elephant. We can only see a complete picture when we combine all of the research that has been done, and synthesize all the things we've learned.

Since you bought this book, I know that you are already familiar with fibromyalgia. You've probably been researching this illness for years, Googling phrases like, "Why does my body hurt all over?" I'm not going to rehash all of that. After all, you bought this book because you want to get back to living your life, free from the prison fibromyalgia has kept you in–not because you want to be an expert on fibromyalgia! I'm betting that you wish that you knew fibromyalgia in a less... *intimate* way, am I right?

Most of this book will be about how to break free from that prison. However, I do want to make sure that it is built on a solid foundation. There's a lot of misinformation and myths surrounding fibromyalgia, so let's go over the basics.

Fibromyalgia varies from patient to patient.
It's easiest to describe fibromyalgia as a chronic pain condition–but you and I both know there's a whole lot more to it than that! Fibromyalgia doesn't just cause pain; it makes you exhausted, disturbs your sleep, and clouds your brain. Many times it feels like there's no rhyme or reason for what symptoms you experience when–or where–or how bad your symptoms are. Fibromyalgia waxes and wanes, and varies widely from patient to patient. This is one reason that it can be so difficult to diagnose.

There are many other illnesses that show up alongside fibromyalgia, adding their symptoms to the mix: autoimmune conditions, depression, anxiety, digestive issues, headaches, vitamin deficiencies, hormone and neurotransmitter imbalances, various chronic infections, and so forth. These illnesses travel in packs. If you are diagnosed with one, you'll probably end up with several. One of my friends, Melissa Swanson, advocate and author of the popular blog Fibro Warriors ~ Living Life, says that her fibromyalgia has come with 19 "evil sidekicks." I've been diagnosed with almost as many different conditions as she has, in addition to fibromyalgia.

Fibromyalgia isn't new, nor is it rare. Descriptions of fibromyalgia can be found in medical literature from the early 1800s, when it was called "muscular rheumatism." Dr. William Balfour, surgeon at the University of Edinburgh, gave the first full description of fibromyalgia in 1816, and described tender points in 1824.[2] The name was changed to "fibrositis" in 1904, then, finally, to fibromyalgia in 1976.[3] It affects two to six percent of the world's population. Based on a conservative estimate of three percent, and the fact that fibromyalgia is diagnosed more often in women than men, one in 21 women currently suffers from fibromyalgia here in the United States. It affects about one in 83 men. Some estimates have fibromyalgia affecting as much as eight percent of the world's population, which would mean one in every eight women.

Science is making discoveries, but has not yet found a cure.

There is currently no cure for fibromyalgia, but it isn't fatal. In other words, you will die with fibromyalgia, but you won't die from it. And please, bear with me a little longer. I know the question you're thinking right now, and I'll answer it in the next chapter. (Hint: Yes, you can get better, even though there is no cure!)

Although there are cognitive symptoms, fibromyalgia is not a mental illness. It is a real, complex, physical condition. Here are a few things that I find particularly interesting about fibromyalgia, based on the current science:

Fibromyalgia patients process pain differently.

While we don't know why, we do know that the brains of fibromyalgia patients experience pain differently than "non-fibro" brains. This difference can be seen on scans using functional magnetic resonance imaging (fMRIs).[4] We experience pain more easily, and different parts of our brains are activated in response to that pain. When talking about this study, Daniel Clauw, MD, said, "In the [fibromyalgia] patients... mild pressure also produced measurable brain responses in areas that process the sensation of pain. But the same kind of brain responses weren't seen in control subjects until the pressure on their thumb was more than doubled." To put it another way, fibromyalgia patients experienced the same pain sensation as their healthy counterparts at only half the amount of pressure.

Fibromyalgia causes hyperalgesia, an increased pain response to painful stimuli. This, for example, makes a pinprick feel like someone has stabbed you with a knife. Fibromyalgia also causes allodynia, which is pain in response to normally non-painful contact, like a hug or wearing clothes. Since we can't walk around naked all the time, this can be a bit of a problem!

Some fibromyalgia patients have extra nerve fibers in their hands.

In June 2013, *Pain Medicine* published a study that prompted the "mystery is solved" article I mentioned earlier. After taking biopsies from the hands of both fibromyalgia patients and healthy control subjects, researchers found, "an enormous increase in sensory nerve fibers at specific sites within the blood vessels of the skin in the palms of the hands."[5] Dr. Frank L. Rice, lead researcher on this study said, "...the pathology discovered among these shunts in the hands could be interfering with blood flow to the muscles throughout the body. This mismanaged blood flow could be the source of muscular pain and achiness, and the sense of fatigue–which are thought to be due to a build-up of lactic acid and low levels of inflammation [in] fibromyalgia patients. This, in turn, could contribute to the hyperactivity in the brain."[6] In other words, the additional nerve fibers in the hands of these fibromyalgia patients could be interfering with blood flow. The mismanaged blood flow could be causing pain, fatigue, and inflammation, which could lead to a brain stuck on high alert.

Fibromyalgia patients may have mitochondrial dysfunction.

Think of your mitochondria as the batteries inside the cells of your body. Their primary function is to generate energy for your cells in the form of adenosine triphosphate (ATP). A small study in 2013 discovered that fibromyalgia patients have less ATP, Coenzyme Q10, and mitochondrial DNA than their healthy counterparts.[7] Another study in 2015 showed "significant mitochondrial dysfunction with reduced mitochondrial chain activities and bioenergetics levels and increased levels of oxidative stress" in skin biopsies from fibromyalgia patients.[8] If you've ever felt like your whole body was exhausted, or that you ran out of energy too quickly, this could be why!

***Most fibromyalgia patients have a
straight neck or reverse curve.***

When looking at neck x-rays of fibromyalgia
patients, rheumatologist Dr. Robert S. Katz
discovered that 90% of them did not have a
normal forward curve.[9] I find this particularly
interesting because doctors have always
commented on how straight my neck is. Having
a straight neck may explain why so many
fibromyalgia patients suffer from headaches, as
well as neck and upper back pain. This may also
explain why more than half of the fibromyalgia
tender points (explained below) are located in
the neck and upper back/chest area.

**There are four primary symptoms
to look for in fibromyalgia.**

While each fibromyalgia patient experiences a
unique combination of symptoms, there are
four primary symptoms that are common to all.

1. Widespread body pain.

When you have fibromyalgia you hurt all over
with no apparent cause. The pain you feel may
move around. Today, your right thigh feels like
someone is stabbing you with an ice pick.
Yesterday, your leg felt fine and your neck and

shoulders felt stiff and achy. No one knows what tomorrow will bring.

Most fibromyalgia patients have sore spots in locations designated as "tender points." These nine pairs occur throughout your body, as shown on the diagram here.[10] That doesn't mean you won't hurt elsewhere. These 18 points are simply sore spots that most of us share.

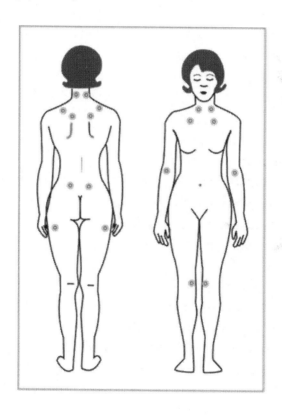

The body pain of fibromyalgia can take many forms. It might be a deep ache, sharp and stabbing, or burn like fire. Under normal circumstances, pain indicates that something is wrong. Rheumatoid arthritis, for instance, results in joint degeneration, which causes pain; this isn't the case with fibromyalgia. There doesn't appear to be anything wrong with our joints or muscles–other than the fact that they hurt! One theory is that the pain we feel is coming from our fascia, the thin sheaths of fibrous tissue that surround every muscle and organ. (Think of the last time you took the skin off a chicken breast. The fascia is that thin, strong tissue just under the skin, surrounding the muscle.)

2. Fatigue.

My biggest fibromyalgia symptom was always fatigue. As one of my clients put it, "I'm so tired that I feel like I have to lie down or I'll fall out of my chair!"

The fatigue you feel with fibromyalgia goes way beyond just being tired. It's as if your body is an old cell phone or battery that can only charge 10%, but tells you it's at 100%. You just don't have normal energy levels, and what you do have runs out quickly!

This particular symptom manifests in different ways for different people. You may be tired, feel weak, unmotivated, have to do things more slowly, or have a lower tolerance for activity. Maybe even all of those!

3. Unrefreshing sleep.
One of the hallmarks of fibromyalgia is the fact that you wake up just as tired as when you went to bed. You might wake up and feel as if someone ran you over with a truck while you were sleeping–only there are no bruises or swelling. Normally, sleep should make a person feel better. For fibromyalgia patients, that just isn't the case.

Pattie Brynn Hultquist, author of the blog *Lupus Interrupted*, brilliantly–and colorfully–wrote about her mornings:

> *"I try to get moving to gather the strength I need to get out of bed... I started with moving my swollen, inflamed, burning/searing red ankles... started moving my hips, purple and black and blue with bruising and oh-so-tender-please-don't-let-the-blanket-touch-them...my arms frozen yet on fire...searing hot burning red, like the sun*

herself slapped them...started my
shoulders turning to roll my bloated,
swollen carcass over the edge of the bed...

"Nothing...NOTHING in the entire realm
of the universe could have prepared me
for what I was about to see...the
horror...I have tears in my eyes just
typing my recount of this morning...I
saw...*takes a breath*...

"I saw nothing.

"My ankles looked like ankles. My knees
looked like knees. My hips looked like
hips. And my shoulders... 'Holy crap on a
cracker, Batman!!'...they looked like
shoulders."

– "Confessions of a Superhero...",
LupusInterrupted.com[11]

First thing in the morning is almost always the worst time of day for us. We are exhausted, stiff, and sore. We can't think, and we hobble around like we're 50 years older than we are, if we can even wake up at all!

4. Cognitive problems.

Fibromyalgia patients refer to the cognitive problems we have as "fibro brain," "brain fog," or "fibro fog." One study testing attention capacity and processing showed that fibromyalgia patients respond in a way that is similar to ADHD patients.[12] You may have thought you were just experiencing "senior moments" a little younger than you wanted, or maybe had ADHD, but this is actually one of the symptoms of fibromyalgia.

Guidelines for diagnosing fibromyalgia are changing.

Prior to 2010, in order to be diagnosed with fibromyalgia, you had to have pain in all four quadrants of your body (upper, lower, left, and right) for at least three months, and in at least 11 of the 18 tender point sites.

Over the last few years, guidelines have been changing. Some doctors are proposing a simple questionnaire that patients can answer to give their doctors the needed information to make a diagnosis. Other doctors object to this method, saying that it's too easy to diagnose patients with fibromyalgia when they actually have a different condition.

As I write this, the American College of Rheumatology has the following list published as the criteria needed for a fibromyalgia diagnosis:[13]

1. Pain and symptoms over the past week, based on the total of:

   Number of painful areas out of 18 parts of the body

   Plus level of severity of these symptoms:
   - Fatigue
   - Waking unrefreshed
   - Cognitive (memory or thought) problems

   Plus number of other general physical symptoms

2. Symptoms lasting at least three months at a similar level

3. No other health problem that would explain the pain and other symptoms

There are a lot of other conditions that can be mistaken for fibromyalgia; your doctor will want to run tests before making a positive diagnosis (see item #3 above). If your pain is primarily in your lower body (legs and hips) you may be suffering from hypothyroidism, for example. Your doctor should also rule out autoimmune conditions, such as lupus or rheumatoid arthritis. These overlapping conditions can make it difficult to get a diagnosis. Most fibromyalgia patients will see four different kinds of doctors over three years or more to get their diagnosis. Nearly 25% of patients will see more than six doctors![14]

I've heard some interesting things from doctors over the years. One told me that if I really had fibromyalgia, I'd be yelling if he lightly rested his hands on my shoulders. This is simply not true, and one of the reasons that the diagnostic criteria were changed. What that doctor was talking about is one of the possible symptoms of fibromyalgia (allodynia), but not the way fibromyalgia presents for all of us.

There is a blood test for fibromyalgia.
Not very many people seem to know this, but there is a blood test that you can take to find out if you have fibromyalgia: The FM/a Test from EpicGenetics. Studies have shown this test to be

99% accurate–as accurate as the tests used to diagnose things like HIV.[15]

In an article dated July 30, 2013, the National Pain Report says, "The FM Test looks for protein molecules in the blood called chemokines and cytokines, which are produced by white blood cells. Fibromyalgia patients have fewer chemokines and cytokines in their blood, according to [Bruce Gillis, MD, founder and CEO of EpicGenetics], and as a result have weaker immune systems than normal patients."[16]

As I write this, The FM/a Test is just starting to be covered by insurance and costs $775.[17] Your doctor can order the kit, draw your blood, and a week or so later, you'll know. If you're having trouble finding a doctor to order the kit, submit a request online and EpicGenetics will have one of their staff physicians review your request. Learn more about The FM/a Test online at: TheFibromyalgiaTest.com.

Fibromyalgia can affect anyone.
Fibromyalgia can affect people of all ages and walks of life, men and women alike. One doctor I interviewed said that her oldest patient was a 90-year-old grandma and her youngest was a 5-year-old girl. Fibromyalgia affects more women

than men, with 75-90% of those diagnosed being women. For the statistics given in this book, I've used 80% as the average of fibromyalgia patients being women.

Based on an internet survey of over 2,500 patients,[18] the average fibromyalgia sufferer is:

- Female
- 47 years old
- About 50 pounds overweight
- Experiencing symptoms for over four years
- Married, with children

A survey of fibromyalgia and chronic pain patients, conducted in 2014 by the National Fibromyalgia & Chronic Pain Association (NFMCPA) and Oregon Health & Sciences University (OHSU),[19] [20] also showed that:

- Nearly half of the patients also suffer from chronic low back pain and over one third suffer from chronic migraine headaches.
- Over one third are employed, with 25% working full time.

- Another third are disabled, with nearly 27% receiving Social Security Disability benefits.
- The three hardest tasks for fibromyalgia patients are: vacuuming or cleaning floors, working continuously for 20 minutes, and going shopping.

The exact cause of fibromyalgia is still unknown.

Right now, scientists and researchers do not know what causes fibromyalgia. There are a lot of good guesses, based on the research that I discussed earlier. Perhaps fibromyalgia is caused by extra nerve endings. Perhaps it all traces back to mitochondrial dysfunction. Perhaps both of those things are caused by something else altogether. Perhaps it's the other way around and fibromyalgia causes them both. It does seem, however, that both genetics and trauma play a role in the development of fibromyalgia.

In the internet survey I mentioned earlier, 80% of the responses indicated trauma or chronic stress as the event that triggered their fibromyalgia. Some examples of these traumatic and stressful events include:

- Chronic stress: stressful job or living situation.
- Emotional trauma: a loved one dying, divorce, losing your house.
- Acute illness: pneumonia, mononucleosis, cancer.
- Physical injuries: falling, motor vehicle accidents.
- Surgery: hysterectomy, C-section, spinal fusion.
- Emotional, physical, or sexual abuse.

In my case, the thing that finally pushed my body over the edge was chronic stress. I worked a very stressful job for nine years. At the end of that time, my body just fell apart–and after some time working through various doctors with various symptoms–I was diagnosed with fibromyalgia.

We believe that genetics is also involved, since fibromyalgia tends to run in families. In addition, some people seem predisposed to develop fibromyalgia. For example, two people could be in two identical minor car accidents. One heals and goes on to live a normal life. The other doesn't heal and ends up with fibromyalgia.

A diagnosis isn't the most important thing.
Clients often ask me what to do if they haven't been able to get a fibromyalgia diagnosis. In some ways, having "the f-word" (that would be "fibromyalgia") in your medical file may not do you any favors. For instance, if you want to buy long-term disability insurance, having fibromyalgia in your medical record gives you an automatic *no* from many companies. On the other hand, if you already have disability insurance and want to take advantage of the benefits, you'll need a diagnosis as proof of your disability.

The bottom line is that the diagnosis isn't what's important. The important thing is getting the treatment that you need to feel better. If you have a doctor who is treating you effectively, having "the f-word" in your file may not matter. If you would like to talk through the pros and cons of this, I'd love to help.

CHAPTER 2
CAN I GET BETTER?

"I feel like I can get better, I just don't know how. I wish somebody would tell me what to do and what works!" – Kimberly

"Healing is a matter of time, but it is sometimes also a matter of opportunity." – Hippocrates

That's the big question, isn't it: *can I get better?* At this point, you've probably been to several doctors just to find out what was wrong. Depending on who you saw, you might have been told, "This is what life will be like now. This is your new normal." Maybe it was even implied that life would be all downhill from here. I want you to know that this doesn't have to be the case! I believe it's very possible for you to feel better than you do right now. I've gotten better and have helped others do the same.

In the spring of 2008, one year after my fibromyalgia diagnosis, I began the process of filing for Social Security disability. I remember the moment I made the decision to file. It was in the evening, and we had company coming over the next day. I wanted to clean the house up a bit so that we would be ready. I remember that I was still in my pajamas; I hadn't had enough energy to really get dressed that day–and it wasn't my first day in those pajamas, either. I was sitting down on the stairs while I tried to vacuum, because I was too tired to stand. It was hard. Everything was hard. I broke down sobbing because all of a sudden it hit me. I couldn't take care of my house; I wasn't even taking care of myself! I remember thinking, "Maybe this is what disability is for."

Fast-forward to September 2010, just two and a half years later. It was a typical rainy fall day in Oregon… and I was walking my first 5k. My goal was simply to cross the finish line. It didn't matter if I was last–which was good, because I was last!–it only mattered that I finished.

I know what you're thinking right now. You're wondering how I did it. How did I get from being disabled to walking a 5k? You're also wondering how much I hurt, and how bad I crashed, when that 5k was over, right? As you read through this book, I'll share with you many of the things that helped me get better. As for the second question, I did hurt afterwards; it took me about a week to fully recover from the walk. Life keeps getting better, though; it only took me about three days to recover from the 5k I walked in 2014.

Here are a few things to consider as you begin your healing journey.

Many factors influence your ability to get better. It's no secret that we're all different. We experience fibromyalgia in different ways and to varying degrees. The two main factors that drive how much you can improve are how long you've been sick, and how severe your symptoms are. Based on my experience with my clients, if you have been diagnosed in the last few years and your symptoms are not super severe, you have a great chance of getting your fibromyalgia symptoms under control sooner so that you can live the life you want to live.

Another factor is you. I believe that it is totally possible to go from disabled to thriving. It isn't easy. It takes hard work and determination. Your doctors can help you, but you are the one who will have to do the work. I'll talk about your part of the job in Chapter 7. How much you improve is directly influenced by your willingness to do the work. Your attitude towards yourself and your illness also plays a critical role.

A "shotgun approach" is your best bet.

You will benefit the most from using a "shotgun approach" to treat your fibromyalgia. What I mean is that you'll get the best results by using more than one treatment method or medication. It would be nice if there was one magic bullet that would get you 100 percent better, but there isn't. You can, however, still get to 100 percent by using 50 things that give you a two percent improvement, or 25 things that help you four percent. If possible, track your symptoms while adding in new treatments one at a time. This way, you'll know what works and what doesn't.

So don't be discouraged when you see slight improvements from each new thing you try. Even little changes can add up to big results over time.

There is no cure, but you can feel better.

As I write this, there is no cure for fibromyalgia. That doesn't mean, however, that you will always have to live with your symptoms as they are in this moment. I believe that fibromyalgia can be managed magnificently–so much so, that it's possible to experience very few or no symptoms on a daily basis. These days, I don't have many fibromyalgia symptoms; I can mostly live like I don't have fibromyalgia. I still have to take care of myself and make wise choices, but it's been several years since I had to say no to something that I wanted to do, or felt at the mercy of my symptoms rather than in control of my life and choices.

Don't give up on the hope of feeling better. If your doctor is at a loss for how to help you improve, find a new doctor. Continually look for ways that you can improve your lifestyle and management of your symptoms. There are so many things that can be done to help you feel better! If you're not sure where to go next in your journey, consider scheduling a consultation with me. I would love to give you some new ideas.

It will take time to feel better.
Even if your fibromyalgia was triggered by a specific event, such as a car accident, your symptoms progressed and changed over time. As you work on feeling better, those symptoms will need time to improve. Being impatient with your body only adds more stress–and more stress means more symptoms. Try to gracefully accept that your body needs time to heal and change.

One of the mistakes I see many fibromyalgia patients make is that they give up on treatments too quickly. It may take weeks or even months before you start seeing improvements. You may need to be on a particular medication or supplement for years before your body recovers to the point that you can start discontinuing them. My doctor prescribed several different medications when I was diagnosed with fibromyalgia in 2007. It was three years before I was well enough that I could start to reduce my medication, with my doctor's help–and discontinuing these medicines was a process that took another three years to complete.

Focus on improving each part in order to improve the whole.
It can be overwhelming to try to treat your whole body at once; there are just so many things that could be going wrong. How can you address everything all at the same time? Instead, I recommend that you focus on helping each piece of your body function as well as possible. This will make you feel less overwhelmed–plus, it's really effective.

A healthy body is made up of individual parts that work together in harmony with each other. We can help to bring our bodies into harmony, by focusing on the functioning of each piece: thyroid, adrenals, nutritional deficiencies, digestion, stress response, quality of sleep, and so on. If you've ever been part of a team, you know that the team wins by having each person play their part as well as possible. And the alternative, having the team depend on a single player who is exceptionally strong–or compensate for a player who is exceptionally weak–is going to result in under-functioning over time.

As I write this, I'm listening to classical music to help my concentration. I'm struck by the similarities between an orchestra and our bodies. Each instrument needs to be playing the same piece of music and to the same beat, or it's just noise. Sometimes one instrument will take the lead and play more loudly than the others. Then, they will trade off, letting another instrument lead. As the musicians practiced, I'm sure the conductor spent time with each one helping them play their part in a way that enhanced the whole performance. You can be the conductor for your body, focusing on the function of each piece of your body, helping it come into harmony with the whole. In the end, when all of your body's instruments are playing perfectly, you will have a beautiful–and healthy–symphony.

You could feel worse before you feel better.
Feeling worse isn't necessarily a step backwards. Depending on the underlying issues you have, and what treatments you try, it may be normal for you to feel worse before you feel better. This is particularly true if you have a chronic infection that needs to be treated, such as Epstein-Barr Virus or a candida overgrowth.

The Jarisch-Herxheimer Reaction, also known as herxing or die-off, occurs when harmful microorganisms are injured or die and release their toxins into your blood and tissues faster than your body can comfortably handle. It can be tricky to find the balance between using treatments that are powerful enough to kill off the organisms that are making you sick, but not so powerful that you are incapacitated by the Herxheimer reaction. Don't be afraid to feel worse so that you can feel better. If you reduce your treatment to the point that you aren't experiencing any symptoms of die-off, then it's a little like trying to bail out a boat with a teaspoon. You're just not making a dent in what's making you ill.

You will want to work with your doctor to make sure that your body is detoxifying properly, give yourself extra rest, and know that what you're going through, however unpleasant, will help you feel better in the long run. Use this quote from Winston Churchill as your mantra: "If you're going through hell, keep going."

Don't give up on becoming pain-free.
A question that I'm asked often is, "Will there be days that I won't have any pain?" This is a tough one to answer because it depends a lot on you. I believe that it is possible. I really don't have fibromyalgia pain anymore, and only need pain medication a couple times a year. Yes, my body has healed, but I'm also very good about protecting my body. I do everything I can to avoid putting myself in a position where I will have pain. I'll talk more in upcoming chapters on ways to avoid pain while still living the life you want to live.

You can't control how quickly your body heals, but you can control what you do and the expectations you have for your body. The better you become at this, the less pain you will have.

The path to success is not a straight line.

Having a setback doesn't mean that you've failed or that you should give up. It just means that you're human; none of us are perfect. It takes trial and error to figure out what makes your body feel good and how to manage your symptoms. Look at life like it's a scientific experiment: test out what you think might be true, learn from what happens, adjust your course, and test again. As long as you're learning something, it is a success.

Think about what it's like to drive a car. You continually adjust your acceleration by how much pressure you put on the gas pedal and brake. You adjust the direction you're going by moving the steering wheel. As you drive, you don't just hold the steering wheel in one position; you move it slightly back and forth to keep yourself on course. Your health is the same way. Slight adjustments to your course are natural, and help you get where you want to go with fewer "incidents."

You may also find that new symptoms and conditions pop up as you work on improving your health. I remember when my doctor diagnosed me with Hashimoto's thyroiditis, an autoimmune condition where your body thinks your thyroid is evil, and tries to kill it. I had spent a full year working hard on my health. I had changed my diet, worked on my sleep, and had even begun to come off some of my fibromyalgia medications. As I was leaving her office, I told her, "You know, I come to see you so that I can get better… but lately it seems like I leave with a new diagnosis every time I'm here! I'm glad though. Knowing what's wrong means that we can fix it." Don't be discouraged if this happens to you. Uncovering hidden conditions, and then addressing them, will only help you get better.

CHAPTER 3
HOW DO I STOP THE PAIN?

"Why do we feel we are bad people for just wanting to be pain free?" - Jennifer

"I'm tired of these heavy drugs and I'm tired of being treated like a drug addict." - Kimberly

"If this is what my life is going to be like–being in this much pain–well... I don't want to live like this." - Chrissy

Malcolm Gladwell, in his book *Outliers: The Story of Success*, talks about The 10,000 Hour Rule. He says that in order to become a master at something, you only need 10,000 hours of practice. While research has shown that it takes more than practice alone to become a master–for instance, you might need a little talent as well–the point behind The 10,000 Hour Rule is one we should take to heart. After 10,000 hours, you will definitely be better at something than you were after 10 hours.

If you think about this rule in relation to chronic pain, it means that your body has gotten really good at hurting.

If you are in pain 24 hours a day, seven days a week, it will take a little less than 14 months to reach 10,000 hours of being in pain. It takes the average fibromyalgia patient three years to even get a diagnosis. (That's 26,280 hours, in case you're wondering. What is that? Ninja level?) If you've spent years–or even decades–hurting, then you are well beyond 10,000 hours! By now, I'm positive that your body has become a master at being in pain.

The earlier you can break the cycle, the better. After all, it will take time to teach your body to not be in pain. You may need another 10,000 hours–14 months or longer–to become a master at being pain-free! In addition, chronic pain is bad for your body. It increases your risk of depression and anxiety, while reducing your sleep quality. Pain can also increase your blood pressure. I know one fibromyalgia patient who was on two different blood pressure medications and still had high blood pressure–until she received adequate pain management. Once that happened, she no longer needed blood pressure medication of any kind. Her blood pressure was simply a symptom of her pain, not a separate problem.

In this chapter, I'm going to give you an overview and some suggestions on how you can get relief from your fibromyalgia pain. It is not meant to be a comprehensive list, but rather a starting place. If you need any help sorting through what might help you most, or want some ideas in addition to what is included here, please consider scheduling a consultation with me.

Treat the three key areas of the pain cycle.
The fibromyalgia pain cycle has three key participants. First, there's the body part that hurts, your leg or hand, for example. Doctors call this soft tissue pain. Second is your spinal cord, which receives the signal from your leg or hand, and passes it on to the third–your brain. Researchers still haven't discovered what causes soft tissue pain in fibromyalgia. Even so, you will find the greatest amount of relief if you address all three areas of the pain cycle.

Let's use the example of a stereo to show how this pain cycle can go awry.

First, you have soft tissue pain. This is like a radio station, broadcasting music. In a healthy person, the nerves in our soft tissue send the right signal at the right strength. You get the right kind of music from the right station at the right volume.

One of the problems within fibromyalgia is that nerve fibers get "confused." Sometimes a painful signal gets amplified between the source and the spinal cord (hyperalgesia). Instead of feeling the prick of a pin, you feel like you were stabbed. In our stereo analogy, this is the radio station that is broadcasting the right kind of music, but at a louder level than all the other stations. (There's a station here in Portland like that. Every time I tune into it, I have to turn my radio down!)

Another way nerve fibers get confused is when a normally non-painful stimulus feels painful (allodynia). Instead of light touches on your arm, you feel as if someone is beating you. In our analogy, this would be like my grandma tuning into her favorite "elevator music" station, and getting my husband's thrash metal instead! Both signals are appropriate at the right time and place, but they've gotten confused, which is problematic.

If that wasn't bad enough, your central nervous system becomes hypersensitive–and this is one of the reasons fibromyalgia pain is so difficult to treat.

In fibromyalgia, your spinal cord can act as an amplifier for the pain signal, turning it up and making it louder as it's passed along to your brain. It's as if your spinal cord thinks that the pain signal isn't getting through. "Hey brain! You're not paying attention. Let me turn this up so you can hear it better!"

As for your brain, it might act like an additional volume knob, turning the signal up, or a tuner, focusing in on a particular signal to make it stand out relative to everything else it is processing. It's as if your brain thinks that the signal isn't getting through the way that it should. "Hey, turn that up! That's important and I can't hear it!" Or, "Tune that station in a little better; I'm getting static!"

The end result of all of these scenarios is that the pain signal ends up getting louder and more dominant overall. This, of course, means that you hurt more than you should. So helpful, right?

In a talk she gave in 2012, Dr. Ginevra Liptan said, "There is still a lot we don't understand about what generates the muscle pain in fibromyalgia. There is some evidence that the pain is from the fascia, the connective tissue around the muscle. So in order to effectively treat fibromyalgia pain, we have to address both the painful muscle tissue and the hypersensitive nervous system."

In other words, we have to use that "shotgun approach" I mentioned in the last chapter. In order to treat fibromyalgia pain symptoms, we have to approach and treat pain in all three of the areas discussed above: the soft tissue, spinal cord, and brain. To quote researchers in Milan, Italy, who studied the pharmacological treatment options for fibromyalgia, "no single drug is capable of fully managing the constellation of fibromyalgia symptoms."[21]

Reduce any sources of pain.
I have a saying, "One good pain leads to another." What I mean is this: when you have fibromyalgia, your body is really good at springing into pain mode. If you stub your toe, your whole body lights up with pain like a Christmas tree. This means that you need to treat any sources of soft tissue or joint pain, reducing anything that could cause you to hurt in addition to your fibromyalgia pain. Your body is, by now, very expert at feeling pain.

I've worked with several women who have had shoulder issues. One of them had a doctor recommend surgery. She was nervous that the surgery would cause a flare-up of her fibromyalgia symptoms. As we talked, it became clear to me that her shoulder was already triggering additional fibromyalgia pain; therefore, I encouraged her to have the surgery. Even though it could cause a fibromyalgia flare–and might make things worse for a time–in the long run, the surgery should reduce her fibromyalgia pain because it will remove a source, or trigger.

If there's a particular part of your body that hurts more often than others, see what you can do to have it treated. You might need to have surgery for painful knees, or work with your dentist to create splints or orthodontia to relieve jaw pain. Dietary changes could reduce abdominal discomfort. Working with a physical therapist or chiropractor could help neck or back pain.

It's important to remember that fibromyalgia isn't necessarily the source of all of your pain. Fibromyalgia can definitely make things worse, but it's a dangerous mistake to think that it's the cause for everything. I know of situations, for example, where patients had their pain dismissed because "it's just your fibromyalgia," when it was really a torn muscle or a rib out of place. One patient I know even went to a different emergency room, in a different town, so that she could be evaluated anew by doctors who didn't know of her fibromyalgia diagnosis. It was only then that the cause of her back pain was identified and treated correctly and adequately. I'm not suggesting that you keep things from your doctors on purpose. What I am saying, though, is that you should make sure that whatever is hurting is assessed properly. You want to make sure that there isn't something else going on, in addition to fibromyalgia.

Take medication so that you can stop taking medication.
Many of us would rather not take medication at all. For one thing, pharmaceuticals can come with some pretty serious side effects. As patients, we don't want to become addicted, feel psychologically dependent, or go through life "drugged" like a zombie. Sometimes, we're made to feel guilty–or worse, like drug addicts– if we ask for medication to help with our pain. For most patients, this results in wanting to take as little as possible, which means we are under-medicating and suffering more than intended.

While these are all valid concerns, it is also true that in order to teach your body how to be pain-free, you must get your pain under control.

This most likely means that you will need some help from pharmaceuticals. You may even need to "layer" with more than one medication to treat the different sources of fibromyalgia pain.

The day I was diagnosed with fibromyalgia, I left my doctor's office with several new prescriptions. Eventually, I ended up on twelve different medications and even more supplements. In a blog article for Invisible Illness Awareness Week in 2011, I counted up 55 individual tablets and capsules in my daily regimen; there have been many times that I took even more than that! Each of the medications that were part of this regimen was an important part of my journey. When my doctor prescribed them, I was having trouble just getting out of bed each day. The prescriptions she gave me helped to calm down my fibromyalgia symptoms and pain, so that my body had a chance to heal. They also gave my doctor and me the benefit of time to uncover and address each of the hidden problems I was dealing with: autoimmune disease, vitamin deficiencies, hormone imbalances, and so much more. Once these other problems were addressed, treated, and corrected, I began to reduce my medications, but it wasn't an overnight thing. I was on some of these medications for six years before I was able to discontinue them. With my doctor's help, I have been able to stop nearly all twelve of those prescriptions. I've also learned which things my body may always need help with, such as thyroid hormones.

I know that you want to be free from fibromyalgia pain and illness, and that includes being free from medications and their side effects. Perhaps you have resistance, like I did, to accepting all the pharmaceutical intervention as a legitimate or sufficient solution. You can always work with your doctor to reduce your medication use once you feel better and your pain is controlled, just like I did. Be open to taking something now so that you can be medication-free in the future. Medication is a tool to use to help you get what you want, just like an ice pack, acupuncture, or stretching. Like all tools, some will work better for you than others. Don't be afraid to work with your doctor to experiment and find the prescriptions that will give you the best relief in the short-term– and your body the best hope of healing for the long-term.

Take pain medication on a regular schedule.

At a recent conference, I learned that researchers conducting studies on pain consider anyone with a regular pain level of four or higher as having inadequate pain management. Take a moment to think about that. If you were to assess your pain level right now, is it above a four? If it is that high or higher on a regular basis, you'll want to rethink your pain management plan. You may need to be more consistent and take your medication on a regular schedule to better control your pain. You may also need to speak with someone about different medication options.

If you wait until you hurt before you take your medication, it's often too late. You simply cannot play catch-up with chronic pain; you have to plan and work to stay ahead of it. Remember that your body is a ninja-level master at feeling pain. Taking your medication on a regular schedule and breaking that pain cycle will help you become pain-free more quickly than if you only take your meds "as needed."

I have chronic daily headaches and migraines, in addition to my fibromyalgia. One day, as I was showing my husband my headache log, he noticed that there were many times that I had a headache, but did not take any medication. He said, very astutely, "The goal isn't to not take medication; the goal is to feel better."

Are you acting as if the goal is to not take medication? Do you hold off until the last possible moment to take something to control your pain? Remember that the goal is to feel better. That may mean taking enough medication on a regular schedule to keep your pain under control.

Think in terms of preventing pain, not just relieving it.

If you take pain medication at the end of a day–after you've done too much, and are in pain because of it–talk with your doctor about taking it at the beginning of the day as a preventative measure. You may still need something at the end of the day, but it will be a whole lot more effective, since your pain would not have spiraled out of control first.

If you find that pain is interfering with your sleep, talk with your doctor about taking something at bedtime. I'll talk more about sleep in Chapter 5. For now, I'll just say that sleep and pain are like Siamese twins, joined at birth and wholly inseparable. Too much pain makes it hard to sleep, and poor sleep makes you hurt more. In my case, switching to an extended release pain medication (one that lasted 24 hours) improved my sleep and reduced my pain levels overall, because it didn't wear off during the night.

If your medication isn't controlling your pain well enough to prevent you from hurting, don't be afraid to talk to your doctor. If she isn't comfortable helping you manage your pain, or has run out of options for you, ask for a referral to a pain specialist. The reality is that there are many options to help manage fibromyalgia pain. If your doctor doesn't give you these options, or does not understand the role of pain in your day-to-day limitations, it may be time to find one who understands fibromyalgia pain and can treat you more effectively. See the chapter on "How Do I Work with My Doctor?" for more insight and practical tips.

Also, consider the lifestyle changes that you can make to help prevent pain. This may mean reducing or modifying your activities until pain is not as active. It might mean choosing a different chair to sit in, or sleeping on a different mattress. Even our clothing choices can impact our pain level. One of my clients, for instance, recently discovered that wearing jeans made her legs hurt. She's switched to softer, more comfortable pants, which reduced her leg pain. What small changes can you make?

Try these treatments for soft tissue pain.

Treating fibromyalgia is never a one-size-fits-all proposition; it's important that you discover what works best for you. To get you started, here are a few treatments that address soft tissue pain, and have worked for me or my clients.

Myofascial Release (MFR): This is a manual therapy, similar to massage, that addresses the fascia. Think of your fascia like a layer of plastic wrap covering your body, encasing each bundle of muscles and muscle fibers. This wrapping can get "bunched up" and that can cause pain; MFR is the process of straightening out your "wrapping." Recent studies have found MFR to be helpful in reducing fibromyalgia pain, if done correctly and by a knowledgeable practitioner. Visit MyofascialRelease.com to find a therapist near you.

Trigger Point Injections (TPI): A trigger point is a knot of muscle that forms when a muscle is tight. While a latent trigger point may not hurt spontaneously on its own, an active one does. Both will radiate pain in predictable patterns when you press on one. For example, there are different trigger points in the neck that can cause your eye, ear, or teeth to hurt. During a TPI procedure, a small needle is inserted into a trigger point. The injection may contain saline or an anesthetic, and may also include a corticosteroid. A "dry needling" technique can also be used where the needle is inserted without using any medications. A TPI treatment's benefit typically lasts one to two weeks.

Topical preparations: Voltaren Gel is a topical NSAID (non-steroidal anti-inflammatory drug) available by prescription only here in the United States. Other topical pain relievers may be custom compounded by prescription, as well. My clients and I have also found relief using magnesium lotion, capsaicin creams, essential oils, and patches, like Salonpas.

Acupuncture: I have acupuncture regularly to help with my fibromyalgia, IBS, migraines, and neck pain. It works wonders at reducing pain in the soft tissue. During a recent acupuncture appointment, while I was lying face down on the table, the front of my right leg started to hurt–in the form of deep, stabbing, electric zaps. My acupuncturist placed one needle in my left arm, and the pain in my leg stopped completely.

You can also use stretching, gentle exercise, heating pads, ice packs, Epsom salt baths, and more.

Calm down your nervous system.

As I mentioned earlier, both your spinal cord and your brain can amplify pain signals. Therefore, treatments that work to calm down your central nervous system overall will decrease the amount of pain that you experience. Sticking with the stereo analogy, these treatments would be like turning down the volume on the radio.

The first FDA-approved fibromyalgia medication, Lyrica (pregabalin), and its chemical cousin Neurontin (gabapentin), work by affecting the chemicals that help to transmit pain signals, such as reducing substance P. (Yes, that's P for pain!) Lyrica and Neurontin also reduce the release of glutamate, an excitatory neurotransmitter.[22] Some research suggests that an overabundance of glutamate may contribute to symptoms of fibromyalgia, such as pain amplification, brain fog, insomnia, and inflammation.[23] I was on Lyrica for several years, and found it very helpful. Another way you can decrease glutamate is to increase GABA, a neurotransmitter responsible for relaxing and calming your brain. GABA is also involved in sleep and muscle function. I've used Kavinace and L-theanine to increase GABA naturally.

Tricyclic antidepressants, such as amitriptyline and nortriptyline, work to "calm" pain transmission in a different way, by blocking NMDA receptors on spinal cord cells. If you're looking for natural alternatives, try taurine, L-theanine, and magnesium.

Another way to turn down the pain volume is to reduce the release of inflammatory substances in the cells of your spinal cord with low dose naltrexone (LDN). I have been on LDN for four years now. It is one of the medications I may never stop taking, because it helps my fibromyalgia, Hashimoto's thyroiditis, and digestion. It does good things for your body, such as boost your immune system, increase endorphins (your natural painkillers), and inhibit activation of glial cells.[24] There have been several recent studies on the use of LDN for fibromyalgia pain. In one study, LDN gave fibromyalgia patients a nearly 30% decrease in their baseline pain levels. LDN, or perhaps the reduction in pain, also improved the patients' general satisfaction with life and their mood.[25]

The only downside to LDN is that you can't take any opioid medications within eight hours of taking LDN, which includes Ultram (tramadol). LDN is generally taken at bedtime, so you can still take your tramadol during the day. The LDN Research Trust has a great website full of information, including a packet you can print out and take to your doctor. Visit them online at: LDNResearchTrust.org.

If you have nerve pain, such as peripheral neuropathy, try these supplements that help protect nerve cells from damage: turmeric, omega-3 fatty acids, and alpha lipoic acid (ALAs).

Help your brain process pain correctly.
"Fibromyalgia brains" process pain differently than the brains of healthy men and women; pain is amplified and processed in ten additional areas of the brain for us.[26] Using the stereo analogy, the treatments below would be like putting in earplugs to reduce noise.

Even though it's fabulous for treating soft tissue pain, I include acupuncture in this category, as well. Acupuncture is very effective at treating fibromyalgia pain.[27] A study conducted at University of Michigan showed that acupuncture helps your brain's ability to process pain signals. One of the researchers, Richard E. Harris, PhD, speculates that "patients with chronic pain treated with acupuncture might be more responsive to opioid medications since the receptors seem to have more binding availability."[28] So acupuncture may even help your brain's ability to utilize your pain medication, making your medication dosage more effective, allowing you to take less medicine to get the same amount of pain relief.

Increasing brain levels of serotonin and norepinephrine will also help. Thanks to popular antidepressants that work by increasing serotonin, and all of their commercials, you may think of serotonin as the neurotransmitter that helps with mood. It will also, however, decrease your pain perception–which is why your doctor has probably already talked to you about taking an antidepressant medicine. It may not be that he thinks you're "just" depressed. Instead, it could be because he wants to reduce your pain sensations!

In addition to helping with energy, focus, motivation, and mood, the neurotransmitter norepinephrine blocks substance P. (Remember, it's P for Pain!) If you look at that list carefully, you'll see how increasing your norepinephrine levels should treat many of your fibromyalgia symptoms: fatigue, brain fog, and pain.

Savella (milnacipran) and Cymbalta (duloxetine), the other two FDA-approved fibromyalgia medications, are both serotonin-norepinephrine reuptake inhibitors (SNRIs).

This means that they block the reabsorption of both serotonin and norepinephrine in the brain. I think of reuptake inhibitors as stoplights, creating a traffic jam of serotonin and norepinephrine "cars." Normally a traffic jam is bad, but in this case, it makes your brain "happier" by leaving more of these neurotransmitters in circulation.

So what happens if there aren't enough "cars" on the road to create a traffic jam? That's exactly what happened in my case. At one point, when I was on three different serotonin reuptake inhibitors–Cymbalta, nortriptyline, and tramadol–my doctor tested my serotonin levels. In spite of all the medication I was on, my levels were "dirt low." (That's a direct quote.) Even though the drugs were preventing serotonin from being reabsorbed, my body wasn't producing enough in the first place to make that "traffic jam." My doctor had me start taking 5-HTP (5-hydroxytryptophan), which is a precursor to serotonin. Today, I take 5-HTP only, no SNRIs. This helps to keep both my depression and my pain well under control.

I do need to stop here for a moment and stress that you work with a doctor on all of this. If you're taking any medications that affect serotonin, DO NOT add in something like 5-

HTP on your own. Too much serotonin can actually create Serotonin Syndrome. If you experience any of these symptoms of Serotonin Syndrome within a few hours of taking a new medication, or increasing the dose of something you're already taking, call your doctor right away or visit an emergency room. I don't mean to scare you, but do want you to be able to recognize the signs: agitation or restlessness, confusion, rapid heart rate, dilated pupils, loss of muscle coordination or twitching muscles, heavy sweating, diarrhea, headache, shivering, or goose bumps. Signs and symptoms of severe serotonin syndrome, which can be life threatening, include: high fever, seizures, irregular heartbeat, and loss of consciousness.

You can also train your brain to tune out pain signals or turn them down. This includes practices, such as:

- Meditation
- Mindfulness
- Breathing exercises
- Biofeedback
- Self-hypnosis
- Relaxation techniques

Consider your medication options carefully.

As doctors have tried to manage pain more effectively, opioid prescriptions have become more common–and so have accidental deaths from these prescriptions. An article from the *New England Journal of Medicine* titled "A Flood of Opioids, a Rising Tide of Deaths" states that deaths from unintentional drug overdoses became the second leading cause of accidental death in 2007. There were 11,499 deaths from overdoses of opioids that year–more than heroin and cocaine combined.[29]

Here are two quotes from that article that really stand out:

"Visits to emergency departments for opioid abuse more than doubled between 2004 and 2008, and admissions to substance-abuse treatment programs increased by 400% between 1998 and 2008…"

"Between 1997 and 2002, sales of oxycodone and methadone nearly quadrupled. …studies have shown a strong correlation between states with the highest drug-poisoning mortality and those with the highest opioid consumption…"

What does this mean for you and me? It means that many of the doctors who freely passed out opioid painkillers to those of us with fibromyalgia in the recent past are now scared. At the Leaders Against Pain training conference I attended in the fall of 2014, a patient very astutely asked, "Are we being treated like drug seekers because doctors are being treated like drug dealers?" Frankly, I think that may be the case. However, I can't blame doctors for being cautious. Research has shown an uncomfortable connection between all of the prescriptions written for painkillers, and deaths by overdose from those same medications.

There are other reasons to avoid the daily use of opioids to treat your pain. Remember the radio analogy? Opioids completely block off the pain signal. This means that your spinal column ends up saying, "Hey! My signal isn't getting through!" and turns its signal up louder. In addition, your brain says to your spine, "Hey! I think something is going on down there; turn that up!" Your brain tries to listen more intently to the pain signal, focusing in on it so that it seems louder.

In the end, you have both your spinal column and your brain effectively turning the pain signal up louder and louder–which means that you hurt more and more. It creates a sort of feedback loop, ending in something like that nasty sound you get when you put a microphone in front of a loudspeaker! Long-term, opioid painkillers could actually make you experience more pain. This is called "opioid induced hyperalgesia"–a fancy medical term for really-bad-pain-caused-by-pain-medications. As if fibromyalgia wasn't painful enough to begin with, right?

Please know that I'm not against the use of opioid pain medication. To quote the Consumer Pain Advocacy Task Force (CPATF), "Allowing people to suffer with unmanaged pain is immoral and unethical."[30] Patients need a wide variety of treatment options, including access to opioid pain medication, when appropriate. I know several fibromyalgia sufferers who have been able to find relief only through the use of opioids. As a patient advocate, and a patient myself, I think this option should be open to us. At the same time, I also believe that it's wise to try other options first, due to the risks that opioids present.

If you and your doctor decide to include opioids as part of your treatment plan, try to keep the dose as low as possible in order to reduce the feedback loop described above. Use them for breakthrough pain–perhaps for your fibro flares–rather than as daily pain management. Why? It's simple. If you use them every day, your body may become used to them and they may not work for when you really need them. As a general guideline, save your breakthrough medication for your ten worst days of the month, in order for it to remain as effective as possible. As a side note: if you're having more than ten days that you'd consider to be your worst, you may need to talk with your doctor and/or revamp your daily routine so that it's more effective for pain management.

Know when it's time to reassess your pain management plan.

One of the first conversations I have with clients is about their pain medication. In addition to the medications mentioned above, like Lyrica and Cymbalta, I recommend talking with your doctor about trying Ultram (tramadol) for daily pain management. It is a milder opioid than medications like Vicodin or oxycodone. This means it carries a lower risk of addiction, dependence, and abuse. It's also less likely to create that feedback cycle I talked about. Tramadol is unique because it's an SNRI, in addition to being an analgesic. This means it will work to relieve your pain by addressing all three of the key areas I mentioned earlier: soft tissue pain, spinal cord, and brain. Tramadol may help to boost your energy (norepinephrine) and your mood (serotonin), in addition to lowering your pain perception.

You'll also want to determine if you're on the "pain roller coaster" by default. Do you wait for your pain pill to kick in, have decent relief for a few hours, and then find that the relief wears off before you can take another pill? One of the ways to avoid this is by switching to an extended release medication, such as Ultram ER, which is taken once a day. For me, switching to Ultram ER made a huge difference in my pain level. Since I took it at bedtime, it was still providing pain relief first thing in the morning. That meant I didn't wake up feeling quite as battered as I did on the immediate release tablets. I also was able to get off that roller coaster, having reliable relief throughout the day. Talk to your doctor to see if switching to extended-release would be a good choice for you.

If you feel like you've maxed out all of the tools in your toolbox–if you've done everything you know how to do and it hasn't helped–it's time to talk to your doctor. It's also time to talk to someone when how you feel physically, day-to-day, begins to get in the way of you being YOU. Even a low amount of pain in the background can nag at you, causing you fatigue, wearing you down, draining you of life. If you are popping over-the-counter pain pills, taking extra naps, and still can't live your life like YOU anymore, talk to someone. Taking some low dose naltrexone or tramadol every day might actually give you your life back!

Whether you're new to fibromyalgia, or are a fibro-veteran, it's never too late to take a new look at your treatment plan. The smallest changes can bring about amazing, life-changing results, just like they have in my life.

I would be happy to help you take an honest look at how your pain is being managed. After living with pain, day in, day out, it's easy to forget what "normal" is in the first place. An outside viewpoint–someone who can see the big picture from a neutral perspective–can be so helpful. You deserve to have a fibromyalgia treatment plan that works for you.

Take it from someone who has been to Social Security disability and back again: You don't have to wait until you lose your quality of life before you to try to get it back!

CHAPTER 4
HOW CAN I HAVE
MORE ENERGY?

"There are so many things that I want to do, but I have to decide. If I do the things I want to do, then I can't do the things I need to do." – Jenn

"I feel like if I don't lie down, I'll just fall out of my chair." – Shannon

Fatigue was always my biggest symptom. For several years before my fibromyalgia diagnosis, I continually felt exhausted at work. I distinctly remember thinking, "If I could just shut my office door, turn off the lights, and lie down under my desk, I would be asleep in two seconds." It felt like even thinking took too much energy! I was like that phone battery I mentioned in Chapter 1, going from fully charged to nothing, incredibly quickly. I think that's why this is one of my favorite subjects to talk about–it was something I had to learn the hard way for myself.

Today, I have the energy to do just about anything that I want to do. I definitely have more energy than I used to, but that's not the only reason. I have also adjusted the expectations I have of myself and make choices that maximize my energy. I've learned how to live with the new needs and energy levels of my fibromyalgia body. I hope that you will look at your energy in the same way: managing it is a matter of making the best possible choices and adjusting your expectations, while gaining energy by helping your body recover.

Making choices means that you do create some control over your daily energy levels. You can't always control the amount of energy your body produces in your mitochondria, but you can control how it's spent–which is the most important part. What we spend our energy on is the stuff of life. You can choose to spend your energy worrying about all the things you can't accomplish, or how messy your house is. Or you can choose to let that go and focus on what really matters: your family, work, friends, loving, living. Your friends and family, especially children, will remember *how you were* at their events more than *if you were* at an event. Were you grouchy because you did too much and are now exhausted and in pain? Or were you happy and supportive, because you chose to go to fewer events but be more fully present when you do participate?

The tools in this chapter are largely about helping you make intelligent choices. It's one thing to choose an activity that drains your energy and makes you hurt. In the fibromyalgia world, these are called "flareworthy" activities. They are the things that are worth doing, even if they cause a flare-up of your symptoms. It's something else, however, to end up in a flare unexpectedly and by accident. All of the tools in this book are about helping you make the best choices possible–to maximize your energy and reduce your pain–so in turn, you can live your life.

Stop the push and crash cycle.

After I was diagnosed with fibromyalgia, I did what I bet you're doing: on the days I felt good, I would do all of the things that I couldn't do when I felt bad. I would do housework, go shopping, visit with friends, and run errands. I did anything and everything. And then I would crash. HARD. I'd be stuck in bed, wearing the same pair of pajamas for a week, paying the price for all of my activity. This is referred to as the "push and crash cycle."

When you break this cycle, you'll end up with more predictable energy levels. You might not get as much done in one day as you do on the "good days," but you'll get a whole lot more done than you did on the bad ones. Things will even out, and find a place of balance. You can then start to rely on your body, knowing that you'll have the energy to commit to lunch with friends, or going to an event with your kids.

Breaking the push and crash cycle is largely about awareness and planning. At first, simply try to be aware of your activities and how they make your body feel. If vacuuming makes you crash on the couch for the rest of the day, make yourself a note to try breaking up the task or asking for help. Be aware of the flareworthy activities too, so that you can plan for rest days around them. If you're not already aware of your push and crash cycle, start there. Once you become aware, you can take simple steps to change it.

If you're feeling a lot of resistance to breaking this cycle, and wonder how this plays out in real life, check out the strategies in Chapter 7. Breaking the push and crash cycle requires that you care for yourself, and know and respect your needs and limits. This may be an area of your health that you haven't explored before. If you need to talk through how this works with someone, let me know. All of my clients have had to work through this idea of pushing and then crashing. We all have responsibilities. Balancing these constant responsibilities against our fluctuating energy levels can definitely be a challenge, and we tend to attribute a lot of meaning to the choices we make, with strong emotions attached. I'd love to help you find your own balance again.

Determine your energy budget.

Managing your energy is a lot like managing your money. You can't spend more than you earn without going into debt. Everything–from food to heat to entertainment–costs money. You can save up for a special event, like going on a cruise, or you can buy it on credit and pay for it later, with interest. The wise thing is to pay as little as possible, which means planning ahead, saving your money, and paying cash.

The same is true for your body. Everything you do requires energy. Most of us are aware that activities like cleaning the house or going shopping take energy, but so do sleeping and healing. You can either plan ahead for your energy expenditures, like walking more while on that cruise, or pay for it later, "with interest."

Energy debt shows up in exhaustion and pain. Just like with money, the smart thing is to plan ahead and budget for your energy expenditures–and reduce your symptoms in the long-run.

In order to live within your means, you have to know your energy budget. This means knowing how much energy your body has available to use, and how much different activities will cost you. This is something that is continually changing and unique to each of us. As a fibromyalgia patient, I've been able to walk in two different 5k races. At other times, I've barely been able to get out of bed to simply sit and stare out the window. Recently, one of my clients realized that she needed to think of doing the dishes as exercise, considering how much it drained the energy from her.

In order for your body to be able to put energy into healing, you've got to leave some energy unused. This is what makes living within your energy budget so important. If you are using every last shred of energy just getting through your day, then your body has nothing left to work with. In Chapter 7, I will discuss more ways that you can help your body heal. I have also created some assignments that will help you determine what your body needs and wants.

Use a pedometer to manage your energy.

A pedometer is my favorite tool for managing energy and fibromyalgia symptoms. It works well to both predict your behavior and as a diagnostic tool to help you discover what has happened. If you're a visual person, you may want to check out the short video I have on my website on how to manage your energy using a pedometer. Visit: MyRestoredHealth.com/book-bonuses.

When I was first diagnosed, I found that using a pedometer gave me more insight to my flare-ups and crashes. I discovered that when my pain and fatigue were manageable, my average daily step count was around 1,000 steps total for one day. To put some perspective on that, it is recommended that healthy men and women walk at least 10,000 steps per day; my average was just one tenth of that.

In general, I found that if I stayed between 1,000-1,500 steps per day, I would feel pretty good–my pain would be under control and I'd have a bit of energy. If I went beyond 1,500 steps and reached 2,000, I would need extra rest the next day; 2,500 steps meant that I would be hurting and need rest. If I reached 3,000 steps, I was in big trouble!

I also learned how many steps different activities would take. Going from my living room to my bedroom upstairs and back cost me at least 200 steps alone. Taking a trip to Costco or Target would be 500-1,000 steps (or more!). And so on.

Knowing all of this allowed me to make better decisions about my activity choices. Managing my steps really was like budgeting money. If I was already at 1,200 steps for the day, and my husband asked me to go to Costco with him, the decision was easy. Another 500-1,000 steps for Costco would put me over my budget. That meant I'd probably hurt the next day and be in bed, wiped out. It became easy to say *no* when I needed to, because I had something concrete to predict how my body would respond to the demand.

Once, early in my fibromyalgia journey, I found myself super tired and sore–way more than usual. I wondered, "What did I do this time?" I looked back at my pedometer logs and discovered that two days prior, I had gone "golfing" with friends. I put that in quotes, because I mostly drove the golf cart. I figured that driving would keep my energy output lower and I'd be safe. Looking at the log for the day of that outing, however, I realized that I had also walked nearly 6,000 steps. That was six times my normal level of activity. No wonder I was tired and sore!

Last fall, I noticed that my step count had gone up by about 30%. I hadn't intentionally tried to walk more or be more active, so this was a fantastic indicator of how well I was feeling. That 30% increase came from me asking my husband a few less times to bring me something while I was sitting and he was in the kitchen. Or choosing to walk up a flight of stairs instead of taking the elevator. Or parking in a space that was easier to maneuver into, but was not right next to the door. It was a natural increase, mostly because I felt better and had more energy. I chose to take steps because I felt like I could–not because I was trying to increase my step count. This was helpful information to take back to my doctor. It told us that the new therapies we were trying at the time were working.

The brand and model of pedometer don't really matter that much. You could get one that is inexpensive and simple, or more expensive and complex. I've also used pedometer apps on my phone. When purchasing your pedometer, look for something that will be easy for you to carry with you. This seems basic, but if it's not on your person, it can't track your steps!

At a minimum, you will want the following features:

- Current step count
- A way to store and view your past daily step counts
- Average daily step count

Other features that may be helpful are:

- Heart rate monitor
- Floors climbed (super helpful if you have a multi-level house!)
- Minutes of activity
- Sleep tracking

I find that the best pedometer is the one that takes the least amount of effort to use. The app on my phone isn't quite as accurate as a standalone pedometer, but it's always with me, and has my averages and history, all stored in my phone. That makes it much more useful than the pedometer that I had to hook up to my computer in order to retrieve and view data. The bottom line is to use what works best for you.

When you first begin using your pedometer, don't try to do anything different. Just let it track your natural amount of steps, so that you know what your baseline is. If that number of steps leaves you tired and hurting, then try to reduce them. If you feel good, you could experiment with increasing. Also pay attention to how many steps it takes to do some usual activities, such as going shopping or to the movies. By knowing your averages, and what different activities will cost you, you can make better decisions on how to spend your energy. This also makes your energy level a whole lot more quantifiable—which will allow you to manage it with more precision—and say *yes* more often when someone invites you to an event.

Here's an example of how you can use your pedometer to plan for activities. Let's say that you can comfortably walk 1,200 steps in a day, and your family wants to go see a movie on Saturday. If you know that going to the movie will take 500 steps, then you know that you can only spend 700 steps in order to stay within your current energy budget and get to do it. That means spending Saturday morning and afternoon reading a book, not cleaning the house.

Discover your body's rhythm.

We all need a pattern of activity and rest. For healthy people, this tends to happen naturally through workdays, weekends, and sleeping at night. However, having fibromyalgia means a need for more rest. It also means that we need to be more deliberate about scheduling rest and activity.

All too often, I see clients who have activities spread throughout their entire week. They feel a bit like Bilbo Baggins, "...thin, sort of stretched, like butter, scraped over too much bread." By having a pattern of activity and rest, just like waking and sleeping, we can give our bodies and spirits time to recover; ultimately, we actually accomplish more.

For years, I have patterned my week to have active days followed by more restful days:

Monday: I work in my office, coaching clients, returning email, and other administrative tasks. I'm using brain energy, but my body is just sitting in a chair.

Tuesday: I schedule meetings outside my office. This means that my body is moving around more, but my brain isn't working as hard. Meeting other business owners over coffee, for instance, doesn't use the same brainpower as writing this book!

Wednesday: This is my self-care day, when I schedule things like massage and acupuncture, or a social lunch with friends.

Thursday: I'm working in my office again, sitting in my chair.

Friday, Saturday, and Sunday: These vary from week-to-week, depending on my schedule. For example, if I have an event on Saturday, I might leave both Friday and Sunday as rest days.

This rhythm of rest and activity, both for my brain and my body, helps me have more energy than if I had the same kind of activities every day. It also helps me to not have both body-draining and brain-draining activities on the same day.

I've also figured out what my best time of day is, and schedule my activities around that, as much as possible. I schedule priority things into the times when my energy and brain clarity are at their best. These may be appointments, writing, speaking engagements, or coaching. It might also be a date with my husband or a get-together with friends; I don't want to leave my friends and family with "leftovers" all the time!

Plan your rhythm so that you can still enjoy your life by scheduling some of your favorite activities into your best times of the day. This is good for both you and your loved ones. It will keep you from feeling like such a prisoner to your illness, and keep your family and friends from feeling like they've lost you entirely. This may mean saying *no* to things you would like to do so that you can say *yes* to what you really want to do. If you've lost touch with what you enjoy doing–or have trouble saying *no*–hang in there. I will talk about that more in Chapter 7.

Make your calendar work for you.
Having fibromyalgia has changed how I schedule my appointments. Before my diagnosis, I usually let other people control when and where things occurred. If you asked me to coffee, for instance, I would let you set the day, time, and place to meet. If my doctor said she wanted to see me in three weeks, I would generally accept the appointment that the receptionist offered. In many ways, I felt like I had little control over my time; I felt like I was at the mercy of other people's agendas and desires.

With fibromyalgia, my energy was limited, so I had to take control of my time. At one point, I realized that I could only have one activity a week outside the house. That meant only one trip to the store, or one doctor appointment, or going to get my hair cut. More than one meant that I would be too wiped out and in too much pain to enjoy my family–or any of the activities I took on!

You might be wondering how I made that switch to controlling my own calendar. It definitely wasn't easy. I had to practice saying *no* and speaking up for my needs. At first, I didn't worry about the appointments that were already on my calendar; I left them as-is. New appointments, however, I began to schedule at better places and times. It was a huge thing for me to tell the doctor, for instance, "I can't come that week, what about the week after?" Or tell a friend, "Let's meet at a coffee shop that has more comfortable chairs."

Here's a technique you can use to start making your calendar work more effectively for you. In this activity, you will create your dream week, based on your own body rhythm, energy budget, needs, and desires. This worksheet is designed to help you see the patterns of your life, rather than day-to-day scheduling on its own. Look at it as a template that you can fit your appointments into. This technique is what I used to help me come up with the pattern of my week that I discussed earlier. Please contact me if you need any help with this.

Step 1: Go to MyRestoredHealth.com/book-bonuses and download the Dream Week Planner worksheet. You'll also find a video that you can follow along with as I explain this process. In addition, grab some blank paper, as well as pens and pencils in different colors.

Step 2: Clear your mind of what you think you *have* to do, and instead, try to think of what you want to do. Take a moment to consider your body's rhythms. Think of how much energy you realistically have each week. What patterns of rest and activity would serve you best? Make notes on a separate piece of paper of the thoughts that come to mind.

Step 3: If you have something in your life that is a regular, inflexible commitment, such as a job, block that out first. I would suggest choosing one color for this type of commitment, so that you know it isn't flexible.

Step 4: Block out your rest times on the worksheet. For example, if you really aren't up for doing anything before noon, go ahead and block out all of the "Morning" slots. If you work full-time and need to rest in the evening when you get home, block out the evening slots. If you have physical therapy at noon on Thursday, perhaps you want to mark out Thursday afternoon and evening to rest and recover. Use a different color to indicate your rest times.

Step 5: Block out any other time you need to take care of yourself so that you feel your best. This could be time for meditation or prayer. It could be physical therapy or a yoga class, massage or acupuncture–or maybe just a hot bath. You may want to choose a different color for your self-care time. If it's a relaxing activity, you might even want to use the same color as for your rest time.

Step 6: Your family and social life comes next. Do you have a date night with your significant other? Are there family meal times? Block these out. Remember to go back to step 4 and see if you need to add any rest time after these activities.

Step 7: Now, look at the spaces. What isn't colored in? Those blank spaces are what you have left for doctor appointments, and everything else.

Step 8: As you look at your Dream Week, does it have any resemblance to your actual calendar? If not, begin scheduling new appointments so that they fit into this template. For example, if you've blocked out the mornings as rest time, don't accept a doctor appointment at 8 AM! Practice saying, "I'm not available at that time, how about the afternoon?" This isn't a lie. You aren't available in the morning; you're resting!

Step 9: Rinse and repeat. Do this activity every so often as your needs change. You will not get this perfect on the first try. That's why it's the Dream Week Planner, not the Perfect Week Planner! It will take some time to get your life to match up to what you've planned. As you try your plan on for size, make notes about what worked and what didn't–and try again.

Another thing to consider, as you put appointments on your calendar, is what I call "transition time." This is the time that you need for activities that isn't being spent on the activity itself. For example, preparing for an appointment, getting dressed and ready to go, driving, mentally switching tasks, the easily forgotten or underestimated details. When you have fibromyalgia, you don't always move as fast or think as clearly as you once did. It takes longer to get ready and out the door, because your body moves slower, or you may need to build in some rest to cope. Activities, such as balancing your checkbook or replying to an email, take longer because your brain is slower. You might even get lost driving somewhere you've been to a million times. By giving yourself more transition time, you can give yourself time to change gears, get your brain and body moving–even get a little bit lost on the way!–and still arrive calm, cool, collected, and on time.

Use a timer so you don't overdo things.
Whether it's true brain fog or just my personality, I easily lose track of time. This is a huge factor in why it's easy for me to neglect going to bed on time, or forget to take breaks when I'm working on a project. A very helpful tool for me is to use an actual timer. By setting a timer, I can fully concentrate on the task at hand. I don't have to reserve part of my brain to pay attention to the time. This works for both physically and mentally demanding jobs. There's a short video about using timers to help you manage your energy on my website at: MyRestoredHealth.com/book-bonuses.

The Pomodoro Technique is a great time management method that makes use of timers. In fact, it's named after the tomato-shaped kitchen timers. (PomodoroTechnique.com, Pomodoro is tomato in Italian.) It's perfect for fibromyalgia patients, too, because you work for 25 minutes, followed by a five-minute rest break. You repeat this work/rest pattern a few times, and then take a longer rest break. Believe it or not, resting your body and mind for five minutes out of every 30 will help you be more productive–while helping you manage your energy.

Pay attention to your pain levels.

Constant pain, even at a low level, is exhausting! I'm not going to say a lot more about pain, since you just read a whole chapter about it. Right now, I want you to remember that you will have more energy if you don't have pain nagging at you all day long. If you've ever lived or worked near a construction zone, think of that constant background noise of machinery. It eventually gave you a headache, right? You probably started feeling grouchy and didn't realize why...until your head was pounding, too. Pain is just like that, sucking the life out of you before you even realize it is happening. If you have any untreated pain, talk with your doctor.

Talk with your doctor about other potential causes of fatigue.

Don't assume that fibromyalgia is the only reason you're exhausted. Many causes of fatigue are very treatable. Make sure your doctor is checking for any other conditions that could cause low energy, such as anemia, depression, hypothyroidism, adrenal fatigue, and more.

Try these supplements to boost your energy.

As I mentioned in Chapter 2, focus on improving each part in order to improve the whole. This means testing for and addressing any nutritional deficiencies you may have. These supplements have been found to be helpful for fibromyalgia patients. They are a great place to start, but this certainly isn't a complete list. Talk with your doctor to see if these supplements, or others, would be good options for you.

Coenzyme Q10 (CoQ10): A 2013 study discovered that the mitochondria of some fibromyalgia patients contain a decreased amount CoQ10 and ATP (adenosine triphosphate).[31] Your cells use CoQ10 to produce the energy your body needs for cell growth and maintenance, while ATP is the energy your body runs on, much like a rechargeable battery. Supplementing with CoQ10 could mean improved energy, due to the role it has in producing ATP. In order to get the cellular energy benefits from CoQ10, your body will need to convert it to ubiquinol, which becomes increasingly more difficult as you get older. Take the ubiquinol form of CoQ10 to get the most benefit.

D-Ribose: This is another supplement that provides key building blocks for ATP. To quote Jacob Teitelbaum, MD, from his book *From Fatigued to Fantastic!*, "Not having Ribose would be like trying to build a fire without kindling–nothing would happen." In a study conducted by Dr. Teitelbaum, participants received five grams of D-Ribose three times a day for three weeks. On average, these patients realized an increase in energy of 45% after just three weeks.[32] In order to avoid a drop in blood sugar levels, and the fatigue that can come with that, make sure to take D-Ribose with food.

Vitamin B1 (Thiamine): In 2013, researchers tried treating fibromyalgia with high doses of thiamine (B1). This study only had three patients, but all three showed significant improvement in fatigue and pain: an average reduction of 56% in fatigue and 63% in pain.[33]

* * *

Managing your energy well is a skill that will make a difference in all of your fibromyalgia symptoms. It will reduce your pain and brain fog, and increase your energy and sleep quality.

It can sometimes be difficult to see "the forest for the trees," as I'll explain in Chapter 8. You're so caught up in just trying to get through each day, that it can be hard to see what you can change to increase your energy. If you find yourself in that position, let's talk. I would love to give you some new ideas.

CHAPTER 5
HOW CAN I GET BETTER SLEEP?

"I wake up so tired; I feel like I've moved furniture all night long." – Shannon

If you don't get quality sleep, you will never feel better. In fact, there have been several studies using healthy college students showing that a lack of quality sleep alone will produce fibromyalgia-like symptoms. In these studies, when students reached deep levels of sleep, researchers would use music to bring the students into lighter stages of sleep. After a few days, the students began to experience body pain, similar to what we experience with fibromyalgia.[34]

On the other hand, if you're in pain, it will be really hard to sleep. I know you've experienced the tossing and turning that happens because you're trying to get semi-comfortable. I know you've also woken up in the middle of the night because of body aches and pain.

If poor sleep makes you hurt, but pain keeps you from being able to sleep, what do you do?

It's a "chicken and the egg" sort of question, isn't it? Resolving the pain and sleep cycle should be tackled from both ends: addressing your pain and improving your quality of sleep. I introduced ways you can reduce pain in Chapter 3, so this chapter will focus on helping you evaluate and improve your sleep quality.

Get a sleep study to check for sleep abnormalities.

One of the first questions I usually ask a client is, "When was your last sleep study done?" Depending on how long ago it was, the study may not have checked for everything that can be detected in today's studies. If she's never had a sleep study, I connect her with a specialist who can check for sleeping disorders and disturbances.

Back in 2006, before my fibromyalgia diagnosis, my doctor sent me for a sleep study, hoping that the results would explain why I was so tired all the time. I went to the hospital, got all hooked up to the mass of cables, laid down, and tried to sleep. Tried to being the operative words there. The next morning, as he helped disconnect me from all the wires, the technician told me that I had zero REM sleep that night. He said that he couldn't see any reason that I skipped REM; everything else looked normal.

REM, or Rapid Eye Movement, is the stage of sleep in which you dream. This occurs approximately every 90 minutes throughout the night. In the six or so hours that I was trying to sleep, I should have had four REM sessions. Once I started to think about it, I realized I hadn't really had any dreams for years. This zero REM thing had probably been going on for quite some time.

A few weeks went by, and I returned to my primary care doctor to get the full results. I got the same information from her–no REM sleep, but no abnormalities found. At this point, my medical team decided that my problem was not sleep-related.

Fast-forward seven years to 2013, after I had been diagnosed with fibromyalgia. My husband decided to schedule a sleep study, because his snoring was disturbing both of us. He came home with a CPAP (Continuous Positive Airway Pressure) machine and his snoring stopped. I thought about writing a blog post titled, "Sleeping with Darth Vader." (Scott's CPAP machine sounds just like Darth Vader's breathing.) The problem was that I still couldn't sleep! I woke constantly during the night, and I couldn't blame it on his snoring! In the morning, I would wake up exhausted, feeling as if I hadn't slept at all. Some of this I blamed on fibromyalgia itself. After all, "waking unrefreshed" is one of the symptoms used to diagnose fibromyalgia! I began to wonder, though, if there wasn't more going on.

At my first appointment, my new sleep doctor told me that I should be getting one to two more hours of sleep at night, now that Scott's sleep apnea was being treated. The moral of that story? If you are sleeping with someone who snores, make them get a sleep study done! It doesn't just affect their sleep, it affects yours too!

I told my sleep doctor about the study I had done in 2006. He said that there were things they didn't test for back then–things that would keep me from getting into REM sleep. He believed that there was more to my story than just the non-refreshing sleep of fibromyalgia.

Sure enough, during my sleep study they learned that I have UARS (Upper Airway Resistance Syndrome). When you have this condition, your airway closes down during sleep–but not completely. Unlike someone with sleep apnea, I don't stop breathing. Instead, it's a little like trying to breathe through a coffee stirrer straw. I'm still getting air, just not very much. When this happens, my brain sends out the crisis message to my body: Warning! Danger! Wake up or you'll die! There's a burst of adrenaline, cortisol floods my body, and I wake up and breathe deeply. This was happening to me FORTY-FIVE TIMES AN HOUR. I was waking up, on average, once every 80 seconds. Whew. That makes me feel exhausted just thinking about it! Can you say, "waking unrefreshed" for a reason?

The treatment for UARS is the same as sleep apnea–a CPAP machine. I love my CPAP because I love good sleep. I won't even take a ten-minute nap without it. I was finally able to come off my last fibromyalgia medication after I'd been using my CPAP for a few months. Addressing any underlying sleeping disorders will definitely help you feel better.

So how do you know when you need to have a sleep study?

If you have been diagnosed with fibromyalgia, and you haven't had a sleep study within the last two years, schedule one now.

Some insurance companies will try to tell you to do an in-home study. Don't let this happen. On the surface, it might seem like it would be a better study if you can sleep in your own bed. The problem is that they can't check all the same things at your house that they can at a clinic. If a wire comes loose during the night, it can't be corrected, and data is lost. In fact, a home sleep study is not recommended for fibromyalgia patients. If your insurance company gives you grief about wanting your study to be done at a sleep lab, just have your doctor call or write a letter that says, "My patient has fibromyalgia. An in-home sleep study is contraindicated in this case."

A good doctor will use the information from your sleep study to check for more than just sleep apnea or UARS. He will check for restless leg syndrome (RLS), monitor your blood oxygen levels, evaluate how much time you spend in each stage of sleep, whether you have bruxism (clenching or grinding your teeth), insomnia, signs of narcolepsy, and more.

Make sure your adrenal glands aren't keeping you awake.

Your adrenal glands are about the size of your thumb, and sit at the top of each kidney. The outer portion of the adrenal gland (the cortex) produces the hormones cortisol, aldosterone, and testosterone. (Yes, women have testosterone too!) The inner part of the adrenal gland (the medulla) produces epinephrine and norepinephrine, also called adrenaline and noradrenaline.

One of the best-kept secrets for getting good sleep is addressing how your body produces cortisol. Cortisol gives you energy, which is awesome when it's time to wake up, but not so great at bedtime–which is the problem we'll discuss here.

Most doctors only check for extremes when it comes to your adrenals, such as Addison's Disease, where your body doesn't produce enough adrenal hormones. A lab test, called the ACTH Stimulation Test, will check your blood cortisol levels to see how your adrenals respond. It's good to have your doctor rule out extremes like this. However, it doesn't give a complete picture of what is happening in your body. It's like taking a snapshot; it only shows the results at a single moment in time, as a response to specific stimulation.

A better test for checking adrenal function throughout the day is the Adrenal Stress Index (ASI). In this test, you collect four saliva samples over the course of the day: first thing in the morning (6-8 AM), noon, 4 PM, and at bedtime (10 PM-midnight). Normal adrenal function is to have high levels of cortisol in the morning, gradually tapering off to low levels at night. You may have difficulty finding a doctor who will do this test for you. In general, I suggest looking for a naturopath (ND) or an MD trained in functional medicine.

It is very common for fibromyalgia patients to have inverted cortisol levels: low in the morning and high at night.

Take a look at my own ASI test results from the fall of 2009 (below). As you can see, my cortisol was WAY below normal in the morning. In fact, when my doctor saw my results she said, "Wow! How do you ever wake up in the morning?" My response was, "I don't!" My usual time to wake up was around noon–the point where my cortisol levels were finally within the normal range.

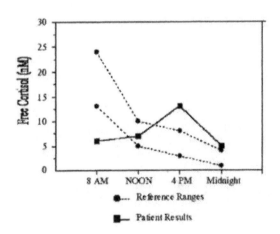

At the same time, I found it incredibly difficult to go to bed before midnight. In my 2009 test, my "midnight" cortisol was actually taken around 1 AM… and it was still above normal! When my husband saw my results he said, "Well that explains a lot!" My best time of the day has always been late afternoon and evening. I often joke that the only way I'll ever see a sunrise is if I stay awake for it!

If your cortisol is high at night, you will never sleep well. Your body is stuck in fight-or-flight mode and feels the need to watch out for danger. As Dr. Ginevra Liptan says in her book, *Figuring Out Fibromyalgia*, "Someone with fibromyalgia awakens feeling exhausted, as if they got no sleep because even in their sleep their brain is awake and watching out for saber-toothed tigers."[35]

Is it possible to turn your cortisol profile back around to normal? You bet it is! Here is my cortisol chart from just over a year later. You can see that I still have trouble with mornings, but the rest of my results are within the normal range, including during the night. No more keeping one eye open for tigers!

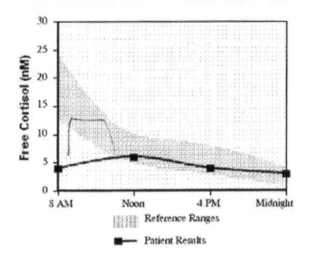

The main strategy I used to turn this around was to help my body shut off cortisol production in the evening. I started by taking a supplement called Seriphos (Phosphorylated Serine). After you receive the results of your ASI test, talk with your doctor to determine what your dose should be. There are three basic ways to use Seriphos:

1. If, like me, you don't get tired at bedtime, take Seriphos in the early evening, before dinner. This will shut down your evening cortisol production, helping you feel tired, letting you fall asleep more easily.
2. If you wake up in the early morning hours, around 2 AM-4 AM, take your

Seriphos at bedtime, around 8-10 PM. This will work to keep your cortisol low during the night, so that your body doesn't wake up trying to be on the lookout for danger.

3. If you have trouble falling asleep AND wake up during the night, split your Seriphos dose in half. Take some before dinner and the rest when you head to bed.

One thing to remember, though: Seriphos controls cortisol but will not help you breathe better. If you wake up during the night because of breathing-related events, you will continue to do so until you treat those underlying sleep disorders.

Increase your melatonin.

Our bodies were designed to get tired when the sun goes down. The darker it gets, the more melatonin your body will produce, and the more tired you will become. At least that's how it's supposed to work.

What happens at your house when the sun goes down? Do you turn on lights, watch television, work on your computer, stare at your smartphone, or even read on an electronic screen? All these things will trick your body into thinking that it's still daytime. Even just eight lux–about twice the brightness of a nightlight, an amount that most table lamps exceed–is enough to interfere with your melatonin production and sleep cycle.[36]

Melatonin isn't just an important hormone because it makes you feel tired; it also helps to reduce pain levels.[37] Fibromyalgia, irritable bowel syndrome (IBS), and migraine symptoms have all been improved using melatonin.[38] Nighttime melatonin levels have been found to be lower in fibromyalgia patients than in healthy subjects.[39]

Taking a melatonin supplement can help reduce your pain, make you sleepy, and reset your sleep clock. If you have trouble falling asleep, try a fast-release melatonin. If you wake up in the middle of the night, an extended-release formula might be more effective for you. If you wake up groggy using melatonin, try a lower dose, or take it earlier in the evening.

You can help your body produce more melatonin naturally by turning down your lights in the evening. If you have dimmer switches, make use of them. You could also use candles, oil lamps, and other sources of low light after the sun goes down.

I have a 7 AM meeting every Tuesday morning. You can imagine how awesome these people must be if I'm willing to get up at 5:30 AM to see them! (Remember my cortisol chart?) To help me prepare for this, my husband and I have instituted "Lights Out Mondays." We turn all the lights off in our living room, light some candles, put on soothing music, and play card games. This helps me feel tired earlier, which helps me get more sleep than I would have otherwise. It's also been a fun addition to our week. Give it a try if you have a similar challenge, and let me know how you like it.

Protect yourself from blue light in the evening.

As I mentioned above, any kind of light can suppress your melatonin production. Blue light, however, is by far the worst. In a study comparing blue and green light waves, blue light was found to suppress melatonin production for twice as long as green light. It also shifted the sleep cycle twice as much (three hours versus one-and-a-half hours).[40]

Amber sunglasses will cut out blue light, and protect you from its effects. Remember the television ads for "blue blocker" sunglasses? You don't just want orange-tinted lenses. You need goggles that block the correct waves of light. I use a pair of Solar Shield "fits-over" sunglasses that I can wear over my regular glasses that only cost me $15.

For years, I've used the Kindle app on my tablet to read in the evenings. Initially, I set it to white text on a black background, thinking that this would reduce the effects a bright electronic screen would have on my body. And it does... sort of. Even with a black background, light is still being emitted. It's as if your electronic device is wearing dark sunglasses; light still leaks through. Set an LCD screen to black, and turn the lights off. You'll notice that it still emits light–and some of that light is blue. If you want to read in the evening, it's better to read from paper (hardcover, paperback, magazine, newspaper). You could also use a Kindle with an E Ink display, since it does not transmit added light; just make sure that your reading light is dimmed. If you're going to read in bed using an electronic device with an LCD screen, or need more light to read by, wear amber sunglasses.

If at all possible, turn off your television and other electronic devices two to three hours before bedtime. This should work to calm down your mind, in addition to helping your body produce more melatonin. If necessary, also cover any electronic screens during the night, such as your phone and alarm clock, to reduce light in your bedroom.

You may also want to re-think the lighting you use in your home. LEDs and compact fluorescent light (CFL) bulbs put out quite a bit more blue light than incandescent ones.[41] Use your LEDs and CFLs during the day, and switch to incandescent bulbs (on a dimmer switch!) in the evening.

Discover what good sleep hygiene means for you.

Sleep hygiene is defined as: *Habits and practices that are conducive to sleeping well on a regular basis.*[42]

Sleep hygiene gets a bad rap. I hear people complaining all the time that "good sleep hygiene" doesn't work for them. I get it. What helps me sleep well may not be the same as what helps you. But sleep hygiene isn't about doing specific things on a professional's checklist; it's about finding out which things work for you, and building a habit of doing them. If you're not getting good sleep and want to try some new habits or rituals, then why not start with those things that sleep scientists have found to be helpful? Just remember, if something isn't working for you, it's time to let it go and try something else!

Here are some examples of what I've found to be effective in my own life and with my clients:

Keep your room cool at night. I keep mine at 64 degrees. At the same time, don't let yourself get too cold, either, or your body will tense up, creating aches and pains from muscle tension. I have a heating pad by my bed (that has an automatic shut-off timer). I often put it at the foot of the bed to heat things up before I crawl in, or warm me up if I get cold.

Go to bed at the same time every day. This will help to set your sleep cycle. Do the same thing on the other side–be consistent about the time you get up each day. Going to bed and getting up are always going to be linked. If you go to bed too late, it will be impossible to get up early and still get enough sleep. If you don't get up until late in the day, it will be difficult to go to bed. Figure out how much sleep you need, set your schedule, and stick to it–even on weekends and vacation.

Eat a protein snack before bed. It can be easy for blood sugar to dip too low, interfering with sleep. Protein before bed can help to keep your blood sugar levels steady.

Avoid anything that might have a stimulating effect in the afternoon and evening. This includes foods, such as caffeine and sugar. It also includes natural supplements, such as B vitamins and tyrosine, as well as herbs we may use for energy, like ginseng or holy basil; and medications, such as those used for ADHD and daytime cold remedies. You may find that other substances stimulate you as well. In my case, the antihistamine used in most nighttime cold medication and PM pain relievers makes me feel wired. Most people feel drowsy when they take these medicines, but I get the exact opposite effect. Make sure to take any medications or supplements according to your doctor's instructions, and communicate with him or her if you suspect that something is interfering with your sleep.

Eliminate as much light and sound as possible. Sounds can distract you from sleep, in addition to the light we already talked about. I sleep with earplugs every night. The ones I use were designed for race car drivers, so not much gets through, not even my husband's early morning alarm. You may wonder what wakes me up in the morning. By practicing the techniques described in this chapter, I usually wake up naturally, before my alarm goes off. On the days that I need an alarm, like my early Tuesday mornings, I have an app on my phone that is loud enough that I can hear it through my earplugs.

Practice relaxation techniques. I have a progressive relaxation CD that I've used for over ten years. Taking time for a hot bath, yoga, deep breathing, stretching, or self-hypnosis can make it much easier to fall asleep.

Clear your mind, as much as possible. Have you ever felt tired, gone to bed, and then had a million things you need to do flood your mind? To combat this, I keep a to-do list by my bed. If anything comes to mind, I can jot it down and let it go, knowing it will be there when I wake up in the morning. I've also found that journaling in the evening can help get things out of my head so that I can let them go.

Prepare for tomorrow today. I find it easier to sleep well knowing that I am prepared for what tomorrow will bring. For any morning meetings I might have, I do all my preparation the day before. I pack my tote with any materials I might need, and set it by the door. When possible, I even make my breakfast the night before. Once all that is done, I can stop thinking about it and fall asleep.

There are no set rules for what your bedtime

routine needs to look like. These are all things that have been found to be helpful, but there is no one-size-fits-all recipe. Experiment to find out what helps you get your best sleep possible. In the "Get to Know YOU" section of Chapter 7, I'll show you a way to track your own experiments and discover what makes your body happiest, which should shorten your trial and error phase!

Give yourself enough time to get the rest you need.

I have always needed about ten hours of sleep. For many years, I fought this. After all, ten hours of sleep takes a good chunk out of your day! I'm a natural night owl. Left to my own devices, I would naturally go to bed around 2 AM. On the weekends or on vacation, when I could get as much sleep as I wanted, I would typically get up at noon. During the workweek, however, I was running on six hours of sleep at most. I was functioning at times on *half* the amount of sleep I needed. It was like someone who needs seven hours of sleep going to work after only three-and-a-half.

Many people underestimate the amount of sleep they truly need because our culture is so sleep-deprived, especially for working-age people and/or parents. Sleep deprivation is a competitive sport, almost a badge of honor in some circles, and the pressure to keep up can soon find many of us telling ourselves that five or six hours is enough. It's as if functioning on more coffee and less sleep makes us better, stronger people somehow. Your body will not keep up with this charade without a protest–especially if you have fibromyalgia.

Do you know how much sleep you need to feel your best? If not, block out your schedule on a weekend or vacation day, and sleep until you wake up naturally. That will give you a pretty good idea of what your body wants. Once you know how much sleep you need, you can start planning for it. This may mean going to bed earlier, or scheduling your day to start later.

Try some supplements for better sleep.
As we discussed earlier, Seriphos and melatonin can both improve your sleep. There are many other supplements that could help you, as well. Here are a few that I use:

GABA (gamma-aminobutyric acid): This amino acid acts as a neurotransmitter that blocks nerve transmission, calming down your nervous system. When GABA is low, you'll feel anxious, hyperactive, and have trouble sleeping.

Since fibromyalgia patients are low on physical energy, the hyperactive feeling may manifest itself as feeling antsy: agitated, fidgety, wired (but still tired), restless, and stir-crazy. GABA is also involved in our pain perception. Fibromyalgia patients with low GABA levels have a low pressure-pain threshold–they felt more pain at a lower amount of pressure.[43] I have used both Kavinace by NeuroScience and L-theanine to increase GABA naturally.

Magnesium: In addition to what we discussed in Chapter 3, this vital mineral helps your GABA receptors function, reduces cortisol, and is involved in melatonin production. Chronic insomnia is one of the main symptoms of magnesium deficiency. Since magnesium needs to be balanced by calcium, talk to your doctor about what amount is right for you.

Iron: If your levels are low, increasing your iron intake will help to reduce symptoms of restless leg syndrome (RLS).[44] Iron overdose can be toxic. Work closely with your doctor on how much you should take, based on your blood test results.

Sleep in a bed that you love.
When Scott and I got married, we bought a split-king adjustable Sleep Number bed. It's

called a "split-king" because it's actually two smaller beds pushed together to make a king-sized one. I often joke that the secret to our happy marriage has been that we sleep in separate beds. In all truthfulness, it has made a huge difference for me to be able to adjust the firmness of my bed–as well as raise and lower the head and foot–depending on my needs, without changing Scott's bed.

I'm not the only one who finds an adjustable air bed helpful. A study published in 2000 reported that sleeping on a bed like mine reduced pain for 95% of the participants and improved sleep quality for 88%.[45] And it didn't just help a little–it helped a lot! These folks averaged 73% better sleep and 32% less pain.

If buying a whole new bed is cost prohibitive, you could check out adding a topper to the mattress you already have.

The important thing is to find something that makes your body say "Ahhh!" when you lie down. There are so many kinds of mattresses you can try: memory foam, latex, innerspring, cotton, air, water, etc. A few of these can be put on an adjustable base that will allow you to raise and lower the head and foot of your bed. If your body doesn't like the bed you're sleeping in, consider looking for a new one.

Talk to your doctor about medications.
If you've tried some natural solutions and still aren't getting the quality of sleep you need, make an appointment with your doctor to discuss sleep help. There are several medications that can be used to correct the sleep problems associated with fibromyalgia.

The first objective in improving sleep on your own is to coach your brain out of thinking it needs to watch out for tigers during the night. Depending on your situation, you may need extra help to silence any racing thoughts that appear when you're trying to sleep. You might also need help calming down your fight-or-flight response, or simply a sedative agent to put you to sleep while you continue to work on improving habits around sleep.

I would love to hear from you with any questions you may have–whether it's tips on how to learn to love your CPAP machine, concerns over medication side effects, or how to honor the two-year-old inside you that refuses to go to bed!

CHAPTER 6
HOW DO I WORK WITH MY DOCTOR?

"I have no idea who to turn to for help and feel very abandoned. It has been hard for me to find practitioners who understand." – Amy

"I feel like I can make decisions for myself now. Before, I felt like all the decisions were being made for me by my doctor and insurance company." – Cyndie

Fibromyalgia is a disease without a home. Technically, it falls under the heading of rheumatology. However, I know very few rheumatologists who treat fibromyalgia. In fact, I know very few doctors of any kind that effectively treat fibromyalgia! This can become quite a challenge when you're trying to find a good doctor. This chapter will help you make the most of the doctor-patient relationship by helping you create your health care team, prepare for your appointment, and communicate effectively with your doctor.

Create a health care team.

Working with health care professionals requires the same "shotgun approach" I talked about in Chapter 2; it's unlikely that one doctor will be able to meet all of your needs. Each type of provider has different training and areas of expertise. Take inventory of this, and create a health care team that fits your unique needs and preferences.

Here are some of the providers that I have had on my team:

- Primary Care
- Naturopathic Doctor
- Neurologist
- Sleep Specialist
- Massage Therapist
- Chiropractor
- Acupuncturist
- Physical Therapist
- Health Coach

As you can see, I've worked with a wide variety of professionals. Some of them favor traditional Western medicine, such as pharmaceuticals. Others prefer a more natural approach, such as vitamins or herbs. Still others focus on biomechanics. A few of these providers are on my team to treat specific symptoms or conditions, such as a neurologist for my chronic migraines. I've found that a mix of approaches and providers give me the best results and fit with my personality and preferences.

What kind of treatment do you prefer? What are your specific medical needs and goals? Do you want to take medication or avoid it? Do you need quick results or can things change gradually over time? Take some time to think through what you want your medical dream team to look like. Once you have that picture in mind, you can go about adding the puzzle pieces you need to create your ideal team.

This is certainly not an exhaustive list, but you might also consider adding these specialists depending on your needs and symptoms:

- Counselor
- Rheumatologist
- Pain Specialist
- Yoga Instructor
- Personal Trainer
- Osteopath
- Gastroenterologist
- Immunologist
- Endocrinologist

As you find professionals to add to your team, it can get a little tricky to juggle who is treating what. Be sure to designate one person as your primary treatment provider for your fibromyalgia. This is particularly important if you are taking any medications, since there can be dangerous interactions. This may or may not be your primary care provider; in my case, my naturopathic physician plays this role.

You will want to be sure that the providers you choose have good communication skills and are willing to be part of a team. You may have noticed that some doctors are better at this than others! A doctor who wants to be the only provider won't be a good fit in a team setting. In short, you want people who can play well with others!

If you want to incorporate complementary and integrative therapies into your treatment plan, make sure to find providers who are open to this. You don't ever want to be in a position where you have to lie or omit something when talking with your doctor. For example, let's say you're seeing an acupuncturist who gives you some herbal remedies. Due to possible medication interactions, you will need to give this information to any doctor who is treating you. You may have difficulty getting the care you need if your doctor thinks that herbs are equivalent to snake oil.

If you want to get better, instead of just holding steady, I would recommend including a naturopathic, integrative, or functional medicine doctor in your team. These physicians tend to have more training in treating and preventing complex chronic conditions. Nearly every time I see a patient get better, they have a doctor like this as part of their team.

It's a good idea to rethink who is on your health care team anytime you feel stuck or like you're treading water. I'm often told, "My doctor feels like she's reached the limit of what she can do for me." I applaud the doctors who are honest enough to admit this. Very few doctors know the best ways to treat fibromyalgia. Another reason you might be treading water is that you have additional undiagnosed conditions. In my case, UARS (Upper Airway Resistance Syndrome) was interfering with my sleep; adding a sleep specialist to my team helped me improve.

Ask for referrals and consultations.
When you are looking to add a health care professional to your dream team, don't underestimate the power of a referral. Ask your

friends and family about doctors that they like. If you have a doctor that you love, ask him or her for recommendations on other professionals. Take advantage of online reviews and social media. One of my favorite things to do is play matchmaker between patients and health care providers. If you live in the Portland, Oregon, area, schedule a consultation with me around this. I'd love to introduce you to some of my favorite people.

Good reviews will tell you what patients appreciate about a particular provider, but take a look at the bad reviews, too. My husband has taught me that negative reviews are incredibly valuable. Often, a negative review will tell you as much about a provider as a positive one. For example, if you're someone who wants to avoid medication and try natural therapies first, this "negative" review may actually be a positive sign for your situation: "This doctor wouldn't give me a prescription. She just wanted to fix everything with diet and exercise."

When you find a provider that you're interested in seeing, ask for a short consultation to find out if it's a good fit for both of you. Fibromyalgia is a complicated thing, but fibro knowledge isn't the only thing that's important. Take into consideration your team's personalities, preferred treatment modalities, communication skills, office staff, bedside manner, and professional interests.

Prepare for your doctor appointment.

Have you ever been a victim of the 15-minute doctor visit? According to the 2010 National Ambulatory Medical Care Survey (NAMCS), over half of all doctor visits are 15 minutes or less; almost 90% are less than 30 minutes.[46] I've enjoyed working with a naturopathic doctor for many reasons, one of which is that her appointments are closer to an hour. Even so, it helps to be prepared. Make the most of your appointment by preparing ahead of time.

When I was working hard to get my fibromyalgia under control, I saw my doctor every three weeks. On the day before my appointment, Scott and I would sit down and list everything we wanted to discuss with her. I would ask Scott how he thought different therapies were working, if he noticed any difference in my symptoms (for better or worse), and if there was anything that he thought we should ask that wasn't on my radar. Often, he would notice different things than I did. For instance, he was more likely to notice the quality of my sleep; if I had a bad night's sleep, so did he! Scott also had a better grasp of my energy level because the more tired I was, the more I would ask for his help.

Creating a list of what you want to talk about–and prioritizing that list–will help you get the most out of the limited time you have with your doctor. In my case, I found that I could usually only get to the first three items on my list, at best, during a typical appointment. That meant I needed to decide which three things were the most important, so we could discuss those first. Otherwise, I'd leave my appointment frustrated and lacking the answers I needed.

I keep a list like this on my smartphone. Any time I think of something to talk with my doctor about, I jot it down immediately. Even without "fibro brain," it can be easy to forget this kind of stuff between appointments. If you make notes as you think of them, it will be easier to prepare. Bring an extra copy of your questions and concerns, and ask your doctor to add it to your medical file.

Create a list of medications, supplements, and health care providers that you can print as needed. I'm sure I'm not the only one who has tried to visualize my medicine cabinet, in order to remember each item and quantity, while sitting in a waiting room! Save yourself the time and stress, and have a list you can print.

Create a document on your computer that contains all of the medications and supplements you take; be sure to include the frequency, quantity or dosage, and prescription strength. You'll also want to include any that you take on an "as needed" basis, as well as any over-the-counter medications. If it's a supplement with several ingredients, try to list those as well. Visit my website to download worksheets that you can use to create your own lists: MyRestoredHealth.com/book-bonuses.

Create another document that includes the names and contact information of the medical providers on your team. Include the primary reason each is a member (for example, what symptoms or conditions are they leading on), and how frequently you see them, including the date of your most recent visit. As you prepare for a new appointment, just print these documents and bring them with you. Your doctor can add them right into your file. At the very least, keep a list in your smartphone or purse that you can refer to. You'll find a worksheet for this on my website as well.

If you've tried medications and therapies that didn't work–or had a bad reaction to some–

include those on your list, as well. If you ever decide to go to a new doctor, these documents will make it really easy for your new doctor to see all of your history, what's working, and what isn't. This information is also helpful if your insurance company has a step therapy policy. Step therapy is also known as a "fail first" policy, because often, insurance companies won't cover more expensive alternatives until a less expensive one fails to help you.

Be honest with your doctor about your challenges.

I've always been a pretty positive and upbeat person. This has served me well for most of my life. Remember me telling you about being diagnosed with UARS and needing to use a CPAP machine? My first thought when that happened was literally, "Oh yay! Now I can talk to my clients about what it's really like to use a CPAP!" Not only was I relieved that there was an underlying cause of my sleep difficulty, after many years of struggle, but I was empowered and hopeful that the struggle would soon be over.

Normally, my positivity is a helpful trait. It keeps me hopeful and focused on the solutions, instead of the problem. When my fibromyalgia diagnosis was new, however, that positivity bias also tricked me into minimizing how much my illness was affecting my life, and settling for a new normal that was far less than I would later achieve.

In my appointments, I would tell my doctor things like:

- I was able to go to Costco this week.
- I've had less pain.
- My headaches are better.

Unfortunately, those statements, without context, didn't really capture the reality of my life. Here's what was actually happening in each of those three statements:

- I went to Costco, but it was the only time I left my house this week. It was the only day that I bathed and put on clothes. The rest of the week, I just stayed in my pajamas–the same pair of pajamas. Plus, I was in extra pain and thoroughly exhausted for the rest of the week because I went shopping one time.
- My pain was only a 6 on a scale of 1-10, instead of a 7.

- Instead of having a migraine every day, it was only a couple of times this week. On the other days, I still had a level 6 headache–it just wasn't a migraine.

You can see that what I told my doctor painted a very different picture from what was actually happening, or at the very least, allowed her to interpret my statements to mean my challenges were resolved. Telling your doctors what you think they want to hear–whether it's because you don't want to make them feel bad or because you feel bad that you haven't improved–does you zero favors. In fact, it will keep you from getting better because your doctors don't have a clear picture of your symptoms and can't adjust their treatment protocols accordingly. They think that what they've told you to do is working.

Another reason to be brutally honest is that if you ever need to file for disability, the truth needs to be in your medical records. I learned this the hard way. In 2008, I filed for Social Security disability (SSDI). The first group of statements made it look like I was healthier than I really was. This made my case a whole lot harder to prove. In fact, the folks who were helping me file for SSDI dropped me as a client because there wasn't enough "medical evidence" showing that I was disabled. (In the end, it didn't matter too much, anyway; by the time I saw a judge, I was so much better that I no longer qualified.)

Don't exaggerate your pain or symptoms, but don't make light of them either. Scott often comes to my appointments with me. Sometimes, I think my doctor believes his reporting of my pain and symptoms more than my own. I think it's because he is better able to describe how my pain interferes with my life. It's hard to be accurate about something as subjective as pain. Many clients ask me, "When my pain is at a six, that would be a nine or ten for someone else. How do I report this to my doctor?" Right now, there is no way to have a standardized system of reporting pain. The important thing is that you use the same scale for yourself and be as specific as possible about how that pain affects your life. Don't try to compare what you're feeling with anyone else. Whether your pain tolerance is greater or lesser than average, the goal is to achieve pain control that allows you to pursue the activities you want in your life. Be direct and honest about where there is a gap; it is your doctor's responsibility to help you.

As much as possible, use numbers and

quantities. Be as specific as you can. Here are a few examples:

"I can only stand for 15 minutes." vs. "I can't stand for very long."

"I can only lift ten pounds." vs. "I can't lift very much."

"I can only concentrate long enough to read for an hour." vs. "I have trouble concentrating."

Especially if your doctor (or other health provider) sees you as "high functioning," there is also a chance that your concerns could be minimized or belittled, or you may be encouraged to settle for less treatment and "cope" with a new normal. Consider what happens when you go to a restaurant. Would you tolerate a favorite dish that is prepared with too much or too little spice instead of visiting a restaurant where you are allowed to state your preferences when you order, or perhaps even makes it "by default" the way you prefer it? Think twice about allowing your providers to coach you out of feeling your best.

A pain and symptom diary can be a great way to provide your doctor with specific feedback. Every time I visit my neurologist, I turn in a headache diary. She makes a copy and adds it to my medical record. This daily reporting of pain levels and symptoms will show your doctor the progress you may (or may not!) be making over time. It also gives more weight to your reporting and provides the specifics I mentioned above. If you say that you're at a pain level of eight at your appointment, your doctor might think that you're just having a bad day. If your doctor looks at a pain diary and can see that you've been at an eight for the last three weeks, this tells her something totally different. Visit my website for a pain diary like the one I use with my doctor: MyRestoredHealth.com/book-bonuses.

If you need to, fire your doctor!
Make it your priority to find providers who will listen to what you have to say and show you the respect you deserve. This is far more valuable than an expert who has a lot of knowledge but doesn't listen to you about your specific issues and needs. Doctors who talk down to you or imply that fibromyalgia is a mental illness–or worse, a fake illness–aren't worth your time or money. I cannot tell you how many times I've heard about doctors who "don't believe" in fibromyalgia. You deserve better than that! If this sounds like your doctor, fire him or her, and find a new one.

I often say that we should treat doctors like we do restaurants.

Imagine this scenario:

You show up at a restaurant and stand at the counter while the hostess is on the phone, ignoring you. When she finishes, you tell her that you have a reservation. When you are finally seated an hour later, they don't apologize. It takes another 20 minutes before your waiter shows up to take your order. When your food arrives, it isn't what you ordered, and the final bill is several times more than you expected.

What would you do if this happened? I bet that you would immediately tell all of your friends to never eat there! You would probably post a bad review on every social network you could think of; you might even post that review while you're still sitting at the restaurant waiting. Most importantly, you don't ever go back!

Yet this exact scenario happens at the doctor's office all the time.

Does this look familiar?

You show up at your doctor's office and stand at the counter while the receptionist is on the phone, ignoring you. When she finishes, you tell her that you have an appointment. An hour later, when you are finally escorted to an exam room, they don't apologize. It takes another 20 minutes before your doctor finally comes into the room. She interrupts you before you can finish your first sentence, writes a prescription, orders lab tests, and walks out the door, leaving you wondering what just happened. You don't want to take medication and don't understand why you need the tests. When you get the bill for your visit and labs–and pick up your prescription–you end up owing more than you expected.

Instead of writing a bad review and not going back to that doctor, most patients think, "Well, she must know best, so I'll do what she says and make another appointment."

As I was researching some of the statistics in this chapter, I ran across this information found in Kaiser Health News:

"A 1999 study of 29 family physician practices found that doctors let patients speak for only 23 seconds before redirecting them; only one in four patients got to finish their statement. A University of South Carolina study in 2001 found primary care patients were interrupted after 12 seconds, if not by the health care provider then by a beeper or a knock on the door."[47]

Let me remind you that your doctor works for you. I believe that we need to vote with our money, time, and opinions. The next time you have a bad doctor experience, treat it like a bad restaurant–post a review and don't go back! By doing this, we can change the face of health care. Bad doctors will go out of business and good doctors will thrive.

Be your own best advocate.
An advocate is, "a person who pleads for or on behalf of another."[48] There isn't anyone who can advocate for you better than YOU can. Only you know what you really feel, think, and desire.

If your doctor suggests something that doesn't feel right, please speak up! In addition, be persistent if there's something that you do want–whether it's a particular lab test or treatment. Nobody knows your body like you do. You know the difference, for example, between fibromyalgia pain and ordinary back pain. You know the difference between being frustrated about a body that isn't working quite right and depression. You know what your "normal" feels like–and if what you're experiencing right now is "normal" for you, or not.

I could tell you story after story about

women who had a nagging feeling that, "something just isn't right," and only through perseverance found or persuaded a doctor who ordered just one more test that gave them meaningful diagnosis and treatment. You might have felt that way yourself before your fibromyalgia diagnosis. Being your own advocate means speaking up so that your doctor can do his or her job and track down what isn't right.

At the same time, be open to your doctor's suggestions. After all, she's the one who went to medical school! Be willing to respectfully engage your doctor about why she may or may not recommend a particular test or treatment. By doing this, you will help your doctor to be more effective. A good doctor will look at your relationship as a partnership. You provide her with information on what you're feeling and experiencing, then she does her job of interpreting those things and presenting treatment options.

If you ever want a second opinion on how to best advocate for yourself, please connect with me. I would love to review your treatment plan and give you suggestions for how you can improve. I may be able to suggest additional tests, supplements, or medications you can talk with your doctor about. I can also give you insight on how your doctor's treatment approach compares with the way other doctors treat fibromyalgia.

CHAPTER 7
HOW CAN I HELP MYSELF?

"If your compassion does not include yourself, it is incomplete." – *Jack Kornfield*

Self-care has been defined as:
The care of oneself without medical, professional, or other assistance or oversight.[49]

This definition basically says that YOU take care of YOU. It uses the word "care" to mean actions that you take.

For me, this definition is both vague and incomplete. It also doesn't say anything about how to actually *practice* good self-care.

I like to define self-care as:

The act of treating yourself the way you would treat someone that you love.

I mean two things with this. First, use the same actions towards yourself that you would use with someone that you love. Buy yourself flowers on your birthday, for example, just like you'd buy some for your mom on hers. More importantly, however, I use the word "care" to mean the emotion and attitude you have towards yourself–the words you use and the thoughts you have. You could substitute "care" for love–self-love.

Most people think that self-care is about what you do, such as spending money or getting massages. It's not really about that. It isn't about eating nutritious food or going to bed on time, either. It's not actually about anything you *do*, but rather about the love that you have towards yourself and how you show that love. Those activities I just listed are all the elements of managing yourself *because* you are practicing good self-care. Self-care itself is something much deeper.

When you wake up in the morning and feel exhausted, stiff, and like someone beat you in your sleep, do you groan and think, "Stupid body! Why can't I have just one day where you're not screaming at me?" Or do you offer yourself a little extra care, grace, and support to make the morning easier?

What are the words that you say to yourself? How do you treat yourself when nobody is looking? Do you offer yourself the same grace and patience that you extend to your loved ones? Or are you critical, holding yourself to a higher standard than everyone else?

All of your actions, from taking your medications to what you eat, will be based on the attitude you have towards yourself. Do you have an attitude of love and compassion, or irritation and disgust?

Forget about The Lemon Law.

I've always had a body that didn't quite work right. My parents like to say that they took my sister to the doctor for repair and me to the doctor for maintenance. She was a daredevil tomboy, who ended up with broken bones, scrapes, and bruises. On the other hand, I was sick. A lot. They took me to the doctor often, just to keep my body functioning.

I distinctly remember being frustrated as a teenager with chronic headaches. I visited a neurologist and heard, "There's nothing wrong with you. Everything is perfectly normal; you just have headaches." I thought to myself, even then, "What is 'perfectly normal' about constant, daily headaches?"

By the time I was 18, I had experienced:

- Surgery to open my tear ducts.
- Tonsillectomy and tubes put in my ears due to chronic throat and ear infections.
- Repeated tests to check my hearing.
- Cystoscopy to check on chronic bladder infections.

- Barium x-rays to check my GI tract.
- Six teeth pulled at once to prepare for a retainer and braces.
- Mononucleosis.
- Numerous other needle pokes and doctor examinations, including the neurologist mentioned above.

I remember praying these words, "God, why did you give me this defective body? If I were a car, I would have qualified for the Lemon Law by now! Can't you just fix me?"

I had the perspective that the "real me" was stuck inside of a defective body, like a prisoner. There was me, and there was my body. Two separate things that were at odds with each other. Most of my life has been spent trying to answer the question, "What is wrong with me?"

Don't treat your body like it's a donkey.
Since I saw my body as something separate from my real self, it was easy to treat her like a donkey that was there to do my bidding. I would push and prod and force her to do what I wanted. In fact, I treated my body just like many people treat their computers or office equipment, "Why won't this darn thing work right? I'll show it who's boss!"

Let me give you a few examples:

- I would often go to bed at 4 AM and get up at 8 AM, getting only four hours of sleep a night.
- I would sit at my computer and work on a project for six to eight hours, or more, without eating, drinking, or taking a break. (This is a temptation even as I write this book!)
- If there was something really important that needed to be done, I would force myself to work all night, just to be sure it was done before the next morning.
- When I felt bad, I often ate "comfort food," such as chocolate, ice cream, sugar, carbs... In other words, when I felt like crap, I ate crap–things that were actually poisonous to my body, due to food allergies and intolerances.
- I would ignore the stress and pain signals my body was sending me, such as headaches, fatigue, muscle aches, hunger, brain fatigue, and emotional fatigue; and keep going "because I had to."
- I would often think things like, "You piece of crap body! Why won't you do

what I want?" Or, "You are so lazy! Why can't you get things done like a normal person?" Or, "This is so stupid! Come on, *think*, dummy!"

Let me phrase these things another way:

- I was forced into sleep-deprivation.
- I was starved and treated like slave labor.
- I was fed poison.
- I was bullied into doing things that I didn't really want to do.
- I was abused physically, emotionally, and verbally.

If I told you that there was someone in my life, like a boyfriend, husband, or mother, who was forcing these things upon me, what would you say? I hope you'd tell me to get the heck out of that relationship! I hope that you'd say that this was a really unhealthy relationship and that I needed to find a new way to live. But there wasn't anyone else making these choices or statements; it was *just me*. I would never treat someone else like this; I wouldn't treat that donkey I mentioned this way! So why was I treating myself like this?

Can you relate?

Learning to love and honor your body, and treat her with kindness and gentleness, brings up all kinds of... stuff... doesn't it? There's a reason you and I haven't been honoring our bodies–we feel that our bodies have let us down!

Remember my "Lemon Law" prayer? "If my body were a car, it would have qualified for the Lemon Law by now."

In a flash of revelation one day, I realized that I was treating my body like this because *I didn't like her.* I would pray that prayer, then go right back to abusing my body, just waiting for the day that I'd die and get a new one. It was kind of a "duh" moment for me. *I didn't like my body, so I treated her like I didn't like her!*

No wonder my body responded by not supporting me the way I wanted her to–and by being as stubborn as a donkey! All of a sudden, I realized I couldn't boss myself around anymore. I couldn't push myself to stay up until 4 AM and expect to wake up at 8 AM. My body expected to be fed regularly in order to perform. Just between you and me, I think the reason I ended up with fibromyalgia was because of how I treated my body for years previously. You might say that my body went on strike; she got my attention, and in the process, got my respect.

Jim Rohn said, "Take care of your body. It's the only place you have to live." He's right; you're only going to get one body–the one you're in right now. You can treat her like you hate her; you can abuse her, push her, prod her, and she will eventually give out on you. Or you can honor her, love her, care for her, give her what she needs–what YOU need–and she will respond in kind.

The fact is, without your body, you really can't do anything. Your body is more than just part of you; she IS you. When you love someone, your hands do things for them; your arms hug them; your lips kiss them; your mouth tells them you love them. It's your shoulder that they cry on; your face that they look at in pictures. Talking to you on the phone isn't enough for the people who love you; they miss your physical presence near them–your body. YOU.

Remember that you and your body are on the same team.
To live your best life with fibromyalgia, it's necessary to pay attention to your body. Take care of yourself, honor your body, and know your limits. Treat yourself the way you would

treat your most cherished friend or family member.

Remember that your body isn't the enemy-fibromyalgia is. You and your body are on the same team, fighting the same enemy, and you need to support each other. Give your body the support she needs, so that she can be responsive to the efforts you make to heal fibromyalgia, so she might again be there for you when you need her.

Have you ever been part of a team activity? Have you played a team sport or been in a drama club, choir, or worked on a team project at work? If so, you probably know that effective teams have several things in common. A strong team consists of people who honor and respect each other, and who practice good communication skills. There is little to no bullying, backbiting, or intimidation. Great teamwork comes from each member working towards the common good, rather than looking out for themselves alone.

This applies to your fibromyalgia journey, and your relationship with your own body.

To have a great team for your fibromyalgia fight, you need honor, respect, and good communication among your team members-you, your body, your health care providers, and your caregivers or support people, such as friends and family. You may find this easy to practice with other people, but with *yourself*? Well, that can be a whole different story.

I know that honoring and respecting your body can be a very foreign concept, especially when you feel like she has turned traitor and betrayed you. Remember, your body is a victim in this illness too. Fibromyalgia is what is causing your pain, fatigue, brain fog, and terrible sleep. Your body wants to be well. She was designed to be able to heal herself, when given the correct tools and resources.

And there's another reason to treat your body with respect…your relationships.

Show others how you want to be treated by taking good care of yourself.
Take a minute and let that sink in: Others will learn how to treat you by watching how you take care of yourself.

Let me give you an example:

A few years ago, I told my husband that I wanted to be in bed with the lights off by 11 PM every night. This meant turning off my computer and starting to get ready for bed at 10 PM. I set an alarm on my phone to remind me when it was time to head to bed. When my alarm went off, I'd often be in the middle of something. This meant that I would turn my alarm off and keep working. My hubby would say, "Hey, didn't you want to be in bed by 11?" "Yes," I'd reply, "but I need to finish this first."

How many times do you think we had that conversation before he finally decided that no matter what I said, I didn't *really* want to be in bed by 11 PM? I was giving the idea lip service, but no actual follow through.

Later on, my husband would suggest, "Let's watch one more episode." (And another, and another...) Was he disrespecting me by suggesting we stay up late? Nope. I taught him that I didn't really need to be in bed by 11 PM. *I was disrespecting myself, so he didn't take my desire seriously either.*

Here's another example I see all the time at restaurants:

Someone goes out to dinner and makes a big deal about having her meal prepared gluten-free. The kitchen makes special preparations to accommodate her dietary requirements. The waiter takes extra care, the manager stops at her table to make sure everything is satisfactory...and then she orders the cake for dessert.

What did that just teach the restaurant

manager, waiter, and kitchen staff? I believe it told them that being gluten-free isn't about food allergies, it's just a fad, and isn't important. The next time someone comes in and orders their meal gluten-free, will the staff treat her with the same respect and care? Or will they go ahead and keep using the same kitchen utensils in the back where the customer can't see, and cross-contaminate her food? Perhaps the second customer will have celiac disease or a bad reaction, and yet it is easy to see where the careless attitude was learned through experience from the kitchen perspective.

Take better care of others by taking care of yourself first.

All of this brings up another important point... *Our self-care habits affect others.*

A perfect example of this is with our children. By watching your example, your children will learn how they should take care of themselves.

You may be able to look back on your own life and see how your own upbringing has instilled in you both good and bad habits or attitudes in this respect. Maybe watching your dad gave you an awesome work ethic... but it means you rarely take time off to relax. Maybe your mom was amazing at making everyone feel loved and cared for… and now you are always the last person to sit down to eat or go to bed because you are taking care of everyone else first.

Society in Western culture doesn't do us any favors, either. We are taught from a young age that sharing is good and keeping things for our own use is bad. We're told that we should always put others' needs ahead of our own. We shouldn't be self-centered, selfish, self-absorbed, self-seeking, and so on. In fact, just now, I looked up "self-centered" in the thesaurus and found the following words listed as synonyms: vain, inconsiderate, and thoughtless.

If you were raised in a Christian home, like I was, there's also the question of what being "a good Christian" means. We hear stories like the Good Samaritan, who gave his money and time to help a stranger, and the boy who gave up his lunch so that Jesus could feed thousands. There's even the verse that says, "There is no greater love than to lay down one's life for one's friends." (John 15:13, New Living Translation) And let's not even start on the challenges presented in "the Proverbs 31 woman." I don't intend to turn this book into a Bible study, but for those of us raised in the Church, this is a big issue worth bringing up to examine how it has influenced even our health habits.

What's a girl to think when she needs time to herself to recharge? What if you need to stop in the middle of the day and take a nap? Or can no longer do all of the laundry, cooking and cleaning yourself? What if working 50 hours a week is no longer possible–even though your salary is only based on working 40? What if you can't give what is required and then some, like your boss implies is always necessary? What if you could be "doing enough" based on fulfilling just the commitment made, not the implicit "above and beyond" that might always feel endless and out of your control?

I want you to know that in order for you to take care of anyone else, you must first take care of yourself. If you've ever been on an airplane, you will have heard the flight attendant say, "Should the cabin lose pressure, oxygen masks will drop from the overhead area. Please place the mask over your own mouth and nose first before assisting others."

When you have fibromyalgia, this is even more true. If you don't take care of yourself first, you won't be any good to anyone else.

Do the "really hard" 90%.

A few years into my fibromyalgia journey, after I'd started feeling better and was able to come off of several of my medications, I told my doctor, "Thank you for helping me to get better." Her response surprised me. She said, "My job is the really easy 10% of telling you what to do. Your job is the really hard 90% of actually doing it. You don't need to thank *me*. Thank *yourself*. You did all the work."

And that's the reality of it. 90% of the medical care you receive comes from YOU. Your doctor may make a diagnosis and prescribe a medication, but you are the one who has to take that pill. Your dentist performs an exam and professional cleaning twice a year, but you have to brush and floss daily. You can go to a physical therapist, but if you don't do the exercises as prescribed, you won't improve.

How well you improve, how good you feel, is directly related to the actions and attitude you have towards yourself.

Consider it your job to get well.

In the trailer for her movie *Crazy Sexy Cancer,* Kris Carr says, "There is no escape. You have a full-time job; you are always at the office of healing."

Once you've been diagnosed with fibromyalgia, you have a new full-time job: to get well. You could choose not to accept this job. You could choose to stay sick, or struggle through yet pretend like there's nothing wrong with you. I'm betting, however, that since you're reading this book, you've already accepted that job. So don't go about it half-heartedly! Give it your all.

If you begin to see that it's your job to get well, what might be different?

For one thing, I bet you wouldn't think that taking naps and getting enough sleep were signs that you were being lazy. If you had a cold or the flu, you'd stay home and rest. You'd lie on the couch and watch bad daytime television. You would know that you needed your rest. Living your best life with fibromyalgia is similar; your body needs rest to heal. (But she might not need as much bad TV!)

You might also begin to see that living within your energy budget isn't a limitation. In fact, it's an opportunity to heal. Every time you spend more energy than you have, it takes away from the energy your body can spend on healing. Sure, overdoing things makes you hurt and wipes out your energy; it also keeps you sicker, longer.

One of my friends recently overdid it and ended up in a bad fibromyalgia flare. She said, "I worry that I've pushed too far and I won't be able to come back from it." You might have thought that yourself occasionally. In my experience, it takes months, or even years, of consistent over-activity to get to a place where you can't bounce back. However, just like with money, spending everything you earn doesn't let you get ahead. Save some energy from your activities, so that your body can spend it on healing.

Even on the good days, remember that you're sick. When you were a kid and had to stay home from school, did your mom ever make you stay home *one extra day,* just to make sure you were well enough to return? Mine did. I always found that extra day the most challenging. On one hand, I didn't have to go to school. I even felt pretty good! But Mom wouldn't let me do *anything* fun! I had to sit or lie quietly. I couldn't go play outside, or hang out with friends. It was like she wanted me to keep acting like I was sick, even when I felt better.

After I was diagnosed with fibromyalgia, I did what I bet you're doing: on the days I felt good, I would do all of the things that I couldn't do when I felt bad...all of them! I would do housework, go shopping, visit with friends, and run errands. I did anything and everything. And then I would crash. HARD. I'd be stuck in bed, in the same pair of pajamas for a week, paying the price for all of my activity. This is the push and crash cycle I talked about in Chapter 4.

One day, as I was talking to some friends about my illness, it hit me. I was having a good day, but *I was still sick!* It was just like when Mom kept me home that extra day. I couldn't keep acting like there was nothing wrong with me, just because I felt good. There were consequences for my actions and I'd been sticking my head in the sand. This was a hard realization that forced me to face the fact that my life was different. I was different.

Say *no* in order to say *yes*.
When I talk to my clients about learning how to say *no,* I generally get one of two responses. The first is, "I say *no* all the time! I don't get to say *yes* to anything in my life anymore!" The second response I get is, "I can't say *no*; I have too much to do!" In a recent coaching call, a client said, "There are so many things that I want to do, but I have to decide. If I do the things I want to do, then I can't do the things I need to do."

Which do you relate to?

The thing is, this really isn't about saying *no*. It's about saying *no–so that you can say yes.* It's about making good choices.

In her well-known blog article, *The Spoon Theory,* Christine Miserandino says, "…The difference in being sick and being healthy is having to make choices or to consciously think about things when the rest of the world doesn't have to. The healthy have the luxury of a life without choices, a gift most people take for granted."[50]

My dad taught me that the hardest thing isn't choosing between good and bad; it's choosing between good and *best*. Living with fibromyalgia means choosing between good and best daily–even minute-by-minute. In the midst of pain or brain fog, we have to evaluate what's best for our families, our bodies, and for us to be as well as possible.

In order to make the best decisions, make them when you are thinking clearly–not in the midst of fibro fog. Here are some steps you can take to help you make better choices:

Review your commitments to see where you can trim down. Is there something you're not 100% passionate about? Maybe the time has come for you to let that go. For more objective feedback, consider having this review with a family member or friend who knows your illness and what you're passionate about. I often help my clients with this in their coaching sessions.

Avoid making important decisions when you aren't at your best. This may mean saying, "Let me think about that and get back to you." This way you avoid committing to something that you may end up canceling. We've instituted a "no major discussions after 9 PM" policy at our house. Scott is a morning person, so he's not at his best after 9 PM. Evening is my golden time (remember my cortisol chart?), so I often forget our agreement, and have to be reminded.

Make some "default" decisions up-front so that you don't have to make them (again) later. When my fibromyalgia was really bad, one of the decisions I made was to only have one appointment per week. Whether it was a haircut, massage, or going to Costco, one thing a week was all I could handle. If something else came up, I knew to either say *no,* or schedule it for another time.

Don't lie, but don't feel like you have to explain. The best *no* response, if you don't want to explain, is: "I'm sorry; I simply can't." It's simple yet still gracious. Sometimes, telling folks that you feel like hell and haven't been able to get out of bed to shower for a week just isn't what you want to do, for privacy or dignity's sake. However, lies will come back to bite you in the butt. "I'm sorry; I simply can't," might mean that you're going to Hawaii, you can't get out of bed that day, or you just don't like the other people that have been invited.

It can be a rather daunting thing to realize that you may never again have "the luxury of a life without choices." There's some grieving that needs to be done–as well as acceptance of your "new normal."

You might find that you need to say *no* to certain foods or activities, so that you can say *yes* to less pain and more energy. You might say *no* to cleaning your house so that you can say *yes* to your kids when they want you to play. You might need to resign from some of the outside responsibilities you've taken on, so that you can spend your energy on your family and your own healing.

You can't get away from making choices, so make your choices count. Making better choices will lead you to a better life.

Ask for and receive help gracefully.
When I was a kid, we had a house fire. Our priest at the time told my mom, "Sometimes the

greatest gift you can give someone is letting them give to you."

I find that most fibromyalgia patients are pretty strong, capable people. This means that it's easy for us to forget that we might need to ask for help!

Sometimes, we don't ask for or receive help because we don't want to be a burden to others. Sometimes, we're in denial over what's happening with our bodies. Often enough, we just forget due to brain fog. It can be helpful to enlist gentle people in your life to remind you kindly that you don't have to do it alone, like our priest did for my mom.

You will do more harm by treating yourself like a donkey. You're also denying people the chance to show you that they love you! This can be especially true for the men in our lives, our Mr. Fix-Its. They can't fix our fatigue, pain, or fibromyalgia, but they can fix things that make our lives easier. By giving him a little direction, you can put those problem-solving skills to work for you, instead of feeling like you have to fight them.

One of the frustrating things that can happen is that our loved ones will ask us in the midst of a flare, "What can I do to help?" At that point, when we can't think straight, all we can say is, "Nothing!" Having some conversations up front, not in the midst of a flare or fibro fog, will help those who love you help you better.

Tell the people you're around most often the signs that indicate you're starting to be tired and in pain. I was once at a museum with a friend who said, "You need to eat, don't you?" I was shocked! How did he know? He could see it by the way I was walking. I hadn't said a word. What are your telltale signs? What can your people do to help you avoid a flare?

Think of where you struggle, then talk with your loved ones about how they can help. During a coaching call, one of my clients mentioned having a hard time keeping up with all she has to do during the week. We discussed how her boyfriend always asks how he can help. I suggested that they sit down together each week to go through her schedule. Doing this will allow him to remind her of upcoming events and commitments when her brain is too foggy to remember. As they discuss her needs together, it will also give him the chance to think of other ways he can help make her week easier.

Be specific. People want to help but they don't know how. Telling folks, "I wish you'd help me!" just creates frustration on both ends. Try saying, "Can you help me put away the dishes? It's difficult for me to bend and stretch to put them away."

Ask your doctor for a handicapped parking tag. Here in Oregon, you have to ask your doctor for the tag; your doctor is not allowed to offer it to you. For a long time, I thought that I didn't need one. After all, I wasn't, you know, *handicapped*; I was only 36 years old! However, I started realizing that I would go places, like the grocery store, then leave if I couldn't find a space close to the door–no matter how badly I needed the groceries! Plus, all of my energy would be gone before I even got to the door in a big parking lot–which left me no energy to do the actual shopping. (Hello, Costco!) After I asked my doctor for the tag, she told my husband, "I'm glad she asked. She really needs this." I don't use it often, but I keep it in my glove box because fibromyalgia is unpredictable. Don't be afraid to get this help if you need it.

Add more joy into your life.
When you live life with a chronic illness, it's really easy to have the joy sucked out of you. You have constant body pain and unrelenting fatigue. You often have to give up activities you used to participate in, simply because your body can't do them. You may be too fatigued, or the

activities themselves cause you pain.

Then you go to the doctor and you're told to give up sugar, gluten, carbohydrates, and caffeine. It can begin to feel like an unrelenting "taking away" of things!

Through all of this, it is really important to remember that life is meant to be enjoyed! Especially as you may have also slowly re-calibrated to a lesser normal before seeking help in the first place. Just because you have fibromyalgia doesn't mean that you can't enjoy your life. You do, however, need to be *more purposeful* about adding joy to your life.

Here is an exercise that I give to my coaching clients to help them get in touch with the things that bring them joy. I've created a couple of worksheets to help you work through this. Before going through these steps, download and print them from my website: MyRestoredHealth.com/book-bonuses.

Step 1: Create Your Joy List

Start a list–in your phone, in a notebook, or on your computer–of all of the things that make you smile, bring you joy, and feed your soul. These can be really simple things or big things. They don't have to cost any money, but they might. Anything goes. If you're using the worksheet from my website, you may even want to post your Joy List someplace visible as a reminder.

It's really important that you do not edit yourself in the making of this list. If you really enjoy gardening, put it on the list–even though right now it hurts to get down on your knees and dig in the dirt. We will tackle how to add those things back into your life later on. For now, just make your list.

This will be an ongoing list that you add to over time. Today, you might have just a small handful of items, but that list will grow. You can use my worksheet for starting your list, but it can also be helpful to have this list in a format that you can carry with you. My clients often use a note-taking app on the smartphone they have with them at all times. That way, they can add to their list anytime they think of something new.

I find that most of my clients are out-of-touch with what makes them happy. They have gotten stuck in a cycle of just getting through the day. That's no way to live a life! Get back in touch with what feeds your soul.

My list contains items like:

- Rubbing "The Belly of Happiness and Joy" (my cat SamSam's big furry belly)

- Taking a hot bath with candles and music
- Enjoying nature by sitting in my living room looking out over the valley, taking a walk, or sitting in a park
- Reading a good book by the fireplace with Sam in my lap
- Getting a facial
- Enjoying a movie or nice meal with my husband

As you can see, some of the things on my Joy List cost money and some don't. The important thing is that they give back to me more than money can buy. These are the things that make everything else, like saying *no* and going to bed on time, worth doing.

Step 2: Figure Out Why and What

Now that you have your Joy List started, let's work on adding those things into your daily life. Look at your Joy List and pick one item to focus in on. You will use this item on a new worksheet for the next few steps.

As you think about the item you chose, identify the why or what that makes you happy. If you wrote down gardening, for example, is it being outside in the fresh air that brings you joy? If so, would sitting on a chair on your back deck accomplish the same thing? On the other hand, if it's the satisfaction of helping something grow, would a few indoor potted plants feel the same?

As you go through your Joy List, use a separate worksheet for each activity. Make notes indicating what you enjoy most about each item. Think about each of your senses: smell, taste, touch, vision, hearing, and emotions. For now, I want you to focus entirely on the positive aspects of the items on your list. We will talk about what makes each difficult in another step.

Here's an example from my own Joy List. Taking a hot bath, with candles & music.

The things I enjoy most about this are:

- Heat from the bath relaxes my body.
- Music also helps me relax, physically, mentally, and emotionally.
- Heat from the bath, plus the Epsom salts, reduce and prevent pain.
- I enjoy the smells of the bath oils and candles.
- The darkened room is relaxing and soothing, especially if I have a headache.
- When done well, a hot bath is a very sensual experience.

- I get a great night's sleep after a hot bath, because I'm more relaxed.
- It's a chance to be alone, with no demands.
- There's opportunity to pamper myself during the bath itself: facial, pedicure, etc.
- Music has always filled my soul, even just on its own.

As you can see on this item from my Joy List, there are many things I've identified that I enjoy that don't have to be done in a bath. I find a darkened room very soothing; it helps my body prepare for bed. I love candles, nice smells, and pampering myself.

As you work your way through this exercise, you will be able to identify things that give you joy that you've been neglecting. Just now, as I'm writing this, I realized that I don't just sit and enjoy music as much as I used to. That's something that I'm going to work on doing, now that I've identified it. What are you going to add back into your life that you have been missing?

Step 3: Identify the Barriers

The next step that you'll take with your Joy List worksheet is to identify what makes the activity difficult for you. This could be physical, emotional, or simply logistical. As you do this step, try to take the perspective of an outside observer. This step is not meant to make you feel bad or guilty! Try to step outside yourself to look at the situation. This is a fact-finding mission.

Let me give you an example of what I mean by being an outside observer. Try not to write down, "I don't have time." That may or may not be true. Remember our conversation earlier about making choices? Instead, write this, "I feel like I don't have time." This is 100% true and captures both your busyness as well as your feelings about the matter.

What is getting in your way?

Let's use my bath example again. I've identified the following factors that make it hard for me to take a hot bath regularly:

- Bath tub isn't as clean as I'd like it to be.
- I feel like I don't have time.
- There's nothing for me to play music on in my bathroom.
- I feel like there are too many other things to do.

- It seems like a hassle to draw the bath, get the towels, soak, and then clean up afterwards.
- I forget that I want to take a bath until it's too late at night to do so without shorting myself on sleep.

As you do this step with your own Joy List, don't worry about how you're going to solve the problem. Simply brainstorm about what is getting in your way. Jot down those obstacles on your worksheet. If you're not sure what's in your way, simply try to pay attention as you go through your life. When you feel some sort of resistance to doing one of the items on your Joy List, ask yourself, "What am I feeling? What is getting in my way? Why?" It's amazing what you can uncover simply by paying attention!

At this point, you should have:

1. Created a list of things that bring you joy and fill up your soul. This is your Joy List.

2. Chosen at least one item and identified specifically why that item brings you joy and fills your soul.

3. Identified the barriers that are
   keeping you from enjoying that activity.

If you don't have all three steps complete, please pause here and do that. The next step will be much easier when you have done both step 2 and step 3.

Step 4: Make Adaptations

When the bathtub needs a good scrubbing before I can take a bath, it's an immediate "no go." If I spend my energy scrubbing the tub, I won't have the energy to take the bath! This is the kind of *physical challenge* I was referring to earlier. If you have items like this, you may need to strategize ways to make the activity easier on your body.

Looking at my bath example, I solved the dirty tub problem by:

- Asking my hubby to clean it for me. Most of the time he does, which is awesome! I have to be careful with my expectations, though, because he might not always want to.
- Finding easy ways to maintain the tub, such as using a portable vacuum to quickly clean out dust and hair.

- Having a washcloth handy at the end of my bath to wipe down the tub while it's still wet and I'm still in it. This helps keep the tub from needing extra scrubbing later.

When I find myself putting off taking a bath because I feel like I have too much to do, or that it's too big of a hassle to deal with, that's a *logistical problem*. Logistics can be pretty easy to resolve once you get clear on what the problem is and make resolving it a priority. An outside perspective, such as from a friend or a coach, can help you spot solutions you may not have thought of on your own.

Here's some techniques I've used:

- Scheduling time for my bath. Yes, I sometimes put "take a bath" on my calendar!
- Set alarms to remind me to stop what I'm doing, and go take a bath.
- Have everything I need for my bath handy, so prep time is less.

As you might have been able to tell from my examples, there are two ways that you can make modifications to enjoy an activity. You can adapt the activity itself, so that your body can physically participate. Or you can modify your expectations–of yourself, others, and the activity itself.

A friend told me once that, "Expectations are premeditated resentments." Do you think it's reasonable for me to expect Scott to clean the tub whenever I ask him? Nope. I don't either. Expecting that is a sure-fire way for both of us to build up resentment! What kind of expectations do you have that are turning into resentments? Try to hold life in an open hand, free from expectations and resentments.

Another example that I love to use, when I talk about adapting an activity that brings us joy, is gardening.

Many fibromyalgia patients find gardening difficult. It can be painful to kneel on the ground, carry heavy bags and pots, and use our hands to grip tools. However, depending on what you enjoy about gardening, it can be adapted in countless ways:

- If you primarily enjoy the sun and fresh air, perhaps you can get the same level of enjoyment from sitting in a chair on your back deck.

- If you love the smell and feel of fresh dirt in your hands, perhaps you could try container gardening. With containers, you can sit in a chair and bring the dirt up to your level.
- If you want to help something grow, then perhaps a few indoor plants could fill your needs.

Sometimes we modify the activity, our attitudes and expectations, or all three.

Step 5: Start working on some "Be" goals

At the end of each coaching call, I ask my clients to set a couple of goals for the week, that I can hold them accountable for. These are small, baby steps they can take towards feeling better. I encourage them to set both a "Be" goal and a "Do" goal. The "Do" goal is what most of us think of when we set goals. It's something that goes on your to-do list; something that you DO. For example: make a doctor appointment for next week.

A "Be" goal is different. You've probably heard the phrase, "We are human beings; not human doings." This is a goal that is about simply *being*. It could be a goal that you set to improve yourself: reading, exercise, learning a new skill. A "Be" goal is also a self-care goal. For example: turn off the TV by 9 PM, and be in bed with the lights off by 10 PM.

Your goals for each week should also incorporate items from your Joy List. This will help you remember why life is worth living, and what it is that you're fighting for.

Get to know YOU.

Honor [verb] – *regard with great respect : Joyce has now learned to honor her father's memory.*

Honor [thesaurus] - *esteem, respect, admire, defer to, look up to; appreciate, value, cherish, adore; reverence, revere, venerate, worship.*

When you have a friend whom you love dearly and want to honor, you do it in a way that means something special to her. For example, you may make reservations at her favorite restaurant, which may not be your favorite restaurant. You might go see a movie with her that you wouldn't choose for yourself. The same is true for your body. Do you know what makes your body happy? Finding that out is your first step to honoring her.

Havi Brooks wrote a magnificent blog article, "The Book of You," about discovering these kinds of things. She discusses a process around writing down the things that you know to be true of you–not true of people in general, but true of YOU–and the things you're perhaps still trying to figure out about yourself. I highly suggest reading her article, if you have a chance.[51]

Here are some of the things I've discovered about myself:

- I need ten hours of sleep each night for me to feel my best; I was trying to function on about six–only half of what my body needed.
- My best sleep comes between 6-9 AM. My body is very jealous of that time; she really doesn't like it when I book that time for things other than sleep.
- My body was tired of rushing from thing to thing. I realized that she wanted (and needed!) to be able to breathe and transition gracefully between various tasks and appointments.
- My body would really like me to pamper her with a hot bath every night before bed.

At first, you might not know what makes your body happy. That's okay. Just write down observations for what you know to be true or what you think might be true. Go ahead and also write down the things you're wondering about–things that may or may not be true about what your body needs. If you need some prompts to get you started, visit my website and download the "Getting to Know You" worksheet (MyRestoredHealth.com/book-bonuses).

Here are some examples from clients:

- If I schedule appointments earlier than 10 AM, it's difficult for me to keep them. Is this true all the time, or only if I have too many in one week?
- More than three hours of training in one day leaves me mentally, physically and emotionally wiped out for the rest of the day.
- In order to keep my weekday commitments, I need to reserve my weekends for resting. Or can I commit to something on an occasional Saturday evening?
- If I take a short nap in the afternoon, my body feels refreshed and I can function better.
- A messy house stresses me out, and makes my body feel like she can't breathe freely.

- I'm less stressed when I can listen to peaceful music during stressful transitions, such as getting ready for work or appointments in the morning.
- Driving in traffic makes me hurt. Don't schedule appointments during that time!
- NEVER EVER EVER EAT CHEETOS AGAIN! (I'm including this one exactly the way my client sent it to me. I love this because it's obvious that her body was speaking very strongly to her and she was listening!)

You might feel silly writing things like this down, but I guarantee that if you don't *you will forget.* Think about that last bullet item and the way it was worded. I don't know about you, but I get the impression that she had eaten Cheetos more than once, and in turn had experienced a bad reaction. Sometimes, we forget what leads to disaster because we don't do something very often. Driving in traffic is like that for me. I very rarely have appointments during rush hour, so I forget how bad it can be. Every time I find myself in bumper-to-bumper traffic I think, "Oh yeah! I hate this!"

Remember, the idea here is to figure out what is true about you and your body, not what "experts" say. You are the expert on *you*. Start listening to what your body is telling you, and you'll become even more of an expert on what you need.

At the same time, don't feel like you have to know how it will all work out. Take my bath thing, for example. My body said she would love a hot bath before bed every night. I have no idea how that will ever happen, and that's okay. This list isn't meant to be a set of rules that you have to follow. Instead, think of these things as simply good information to have. In my case, if my body is feeling particularly cranky, I remember that she likes a hot bath before bed, and I give her one.

Here are some things you can think about, as you create your list of what your body likes and doesn't like:

- What makes you feel better if you're having a bad day?
- What makes you feel worse?
- What causes you pain?
- What brings you joy or happiness?
- What do you regret doing after you've done it?
- What do you wish you could do more of?

- Are there any foods that make you feel good–or are there some that make you feel bad?
- Are there people you hang out with who add to your energy?
- Do you know any energy vampires?
- Are there certain activities that you can do for a small amount of time, but not for long periods?

I suggest keeping your list in a format that is easy to carry with you. Maybe you can use a small notebook, or make a list on your phone. If you can have your list with you, it will be much easier to add things whenever you run across something new.

Once you have some ideas for what your body wants, you'll have ideas for changes you can make, ways to improve your health, and tactics for avoiding fibromyalgia flare-ups. For now, though, just get to know you and your body by making a note of your observations.

* * *

If you get stuck on any of the activities suggested in this chapter, such as creating your Joy List, please reach out to me. Getting in touch with what makes you and your body happy is so important, but definitely not easy. Working with me as you go through this can be very helpful. As a coach, I know how to ask questions that will help you unlock your own answers.

CHAPTER 8
WOULD WORKING WITH A HEALTH COACH BE HELPFUL?

"I'm so pleased to be able to work on my healing with someone who understands and can give spot on advice! I'm glad that I don't have to try to be accountable just to myself–which doesn't really work a lot of the time, anyway." – Eleni

The reality is that most of us know what we need to do to feel better. Actually doing it? Consistently? Well, that's another story altogether.

A health coach helps to bridge the gap between what you *know* and what you *do* by:

- Working with you to identify health goals, such as making dietary changes, reducing pain, increasing energy, and improving sleep.
- Providing accountability for the goals you have set.

- Troubleshooting therapies, by helping you interpret what's working and what isn't.
- Encouraging and supporting you.
- Making objective observations of your actions, behavior, and well-being.
- Coordinating between you and the members of your health care team.

Some health coaches want to focus on things like diet and exercise. I take a much broader approach. My feeling is this: if something is affecting your health, we should talk about it.

I once helped a client buy tires for her car. As a fibromyalgia patient, she was dealing with limited energy and lots of brain fog. This made getting tires for her car an almost impossible task. She was too tired to drive around and get quotes; she had too much brain fog to know if she was asking the right questions or making good decisions.

We spent two months of her coaching sessions working through the process. Her first assignment was simply to identify what places to get quotes from. Then, she called a couple of places and got the actual prices. A few weeks later, she visited the shops she was interested in to see if she liked and trusted the people who worked there.

When she finally got tires on her car, her anxiety went way down, her energy level went up, and her brain fog cleared. The stress of having that hanging over her head had been making her fibromyalgia symptoms worse.

If something is affecting your health, either by action or neglect, think about working with a coach to change it.

We all have blind spots.
A coach can help you see things that you can't see on your own, simply because you're in the middle of it all. You can't see the forest for the trees. Having someone on the outside, looking at the big picture story of your life, is so helpful.

One of my clients mentioned to me in a coaching call that her pain level had been higher for the last few months. Later in our conversation, she mentioned that she hadn't been keeping up on her yoga and mindfulness meditation like she used to. My coach radar immediately perked up! I asked her, "How long has it been since you meditated?" You know where this is going, right? She stopped meditating right around the same time her pain started increasing. I was able to see this right away, but she was blind to it.

In another call, a client mentioned that she had found herself snacking all day, and couldn't figure out why. As we talked, I discovered that her desk faced her kitchen. She was literally looking into her kitchen all day long. She rotated her desk so that she could look out the window, and the snacking stopped.

I often help my clients figure out what therapies and treatment options are working for them. One of the tools I use is a food and symptom diary. With one client, I was able to notice a pattern that every time she ate tomatoes, two days later, she hurt more. She didn't notice on her own, because it was two days later!

Even as a coach, I need someone to help me see into my blind spots. I'm trained. I know what to do, but I'm still blind in places.

It's just something you can't do for yourself.

A good coach will help you make choices.
"Do I have to give up coffee and chocolate to work with you?" Every time I see that question I smile. This is probably the best question anyone has ever asked me. There's a lot in that little question isn't there? It's about finding the balance between feeling better and enjoying life,

in my opinion. By the time you've been diagnosed with fibromyalgia, you've probably had to give up a lot that you used to enjoy. There are things you can't do anymore because they cause you pain or make you too tired. So do you really have to give up coffee and chocolate, too? I know you're thinking it!

The answer is–it's totally up to you.

If you feel like you're drinking too much coffee, then sure, we can work on it. If coffee is something that gives you joy, then heck no! Leave it be–at least for now.

My philosophy is to use the path of least resistance. Pick the low hanging fruit. Start with the easy stuff and build up a habit of success. That may sound trite, but living with fibromyalgia is hard. You don't need more hard things. You don't need more things that you can't do. You need to have some success and to feel like you can do something.

Remember the Tortoise and the Hare? The hare is faster... but the tortoise won the race because he kept taking one step at a time and didn't stop until he crossed the finish line. The race to live a good life is just like that. Keep taking steps forward. As one client told me after we'd been working together for a while, "There came a point where all of a sudden, I was doing the impossible!"

You can do the impossible too. Just take it one baby step at a time.

Working with a coach will help you get better results.

Research studies have shown that working with a coach can result in:

- Lower blood pressure and blood sugar levels.
- Better medication compliance.
- Greater weight loss.
- Fewer doctor appointments.
- Less pain and disability.
- Reduced fatigue, depression, and anxiety.
- Higher quality of life.

Those are some pretty great claims! Let's look at a few of those in more detail.

A study published in the May/June 2012 issue of the *Annals of Family Medicine* showed that, "The more coaching encounters a patient had, the greater their reduction in blood pressure."[52] To quote Thomas Bodenheimer, MD, one of the researchers on the project, "The more telephone calls between a coach and a patient, the better the patient's blood pressure.

It's almost like a medicine; *if you increase the dose of coaching, you get a better result.*" (emphasis mine) This same study showed that patients working with a coach had two fewer doctor appointments per year.

Have you ever found it difficult to remember to take your medication? Working with a coach can help with that, according to a 2015 article in the *Journal of the American Board of Family Physicians*. "Compared with usual care, patients receiving health coaching had a significantly greater increase in the proportion of medications for which there was complete concordance of name, dose, and frequency."[53] In other words, patients working with a coach took their medications as prescribed–in the correct amounts, and at the correct time.

A study done at Miriam Hospital in 2012 found that working with a professional health coach gave better results than working with a peer (someone on a similar journey to yours), or a mentor (someone who has done the journey before you, but isn't professionally trained). In this study, a greater number of patients working with a professional health coach lost more weight than any other group.[54]

In northern California, Kaiser Permanente looked at the impact coaching had on patient satisfaction and quality of life.[55] When patients had at least two sessions with a coach, 68% ate more healthfully; 71% increased their activity level; 79% increased their overall health; 73% reduced their risk of disease; and 83% improved their quality of life.

The bottom line? Working with a health coach is good for you!

Any therapy you choose will work better and you'll get better results; you'll save money on doctor appointments and medications; and you'll have less pain, fatigue, and depression–all with improved functioning and quality of life.

Be selective about choosing your coach.

Now that you've seen the difference that working with a coach can make in your health, you might be wondering how to find a good one. Choosing the right health coach is a decision you shouldn't make lightly. Just like athletic and business coaches have different philosophies and styles, so do health and wellness coaches.

Here are some guidelines to help you make the best choice for you and your situation:

1. Find a health coach who is an expert in your particular illness.

I can't stress how important this one is. If you've been diagnosed with fibromyalgia, want to learn how to live well in spite of your illness, and discover treatment options available to you–only a health coach who understands fibromyalgia can help you effectively.

Not all health coaches focus on helping the same kind of people. If you have fibromyalgia, you don't want to work with a coach who primarily trains healthy athletes. That's a great recipe for ending up exhausted and in more pain!

This means you'll want to choose a *fibromyalgia* health coach. Helping fibromyalgia patients should be their *key focus*, not a service that they've tacked on as a subset of what they offer everyone else.

2. Opt for a health coach who understands your struggles.

Now that you know you want a fibromyalgia health coach, you need to find one who has already gone through what you are trying to overcome. Many of us have become health coaches because we worked with a coach ourselves, found success, and wanted to "pay it forward" and help others find the same success.

This means that if you want to lose weight, find a fibromyalgia health coach who has lost weight themselves. If you want to walk a 5k with fibromyalgia, find someone who has done it. If you want to find healing from fibromyalgia, find a coach who used to be sick who is now living the kind of life you want to live!

By choosing a fibromyalgia health coach who has "been there, done that," you'll have someone who truly understands the struggles you face, can give you practical advice, and who won't blindly accept your excuses. That coach will be able to tell the difference between not doing something because you were in a fibromyalgia flare, versus not doing it because you simply didn't want to.

3. Make sure your health coach is up-to-date on the latest research.

There is so much conflicting information out there when it comes to nutrition, fitness, health, and fibromyalgia–plus, it's changing continually. Even the experts don't agree when it comes to some things!

You want to choose a fibromyalgia health coach who loves research, reading, learning, and growing. If she doesn't, she can easily get behind and end up giving YOU bad information. A coach who loves this stuff can stay on top of the latest research–and will share it with you and your doctors.

4. Decide what type of coaching personality you need for your journey.

As health coaches, we all have different personalities–and as a client, so do you! Some coaches are like drill sergeants, where others are encouraging cheerleaders. Some focus on teaching you how to figure things out yourself, where others offer their own tried and true advice and solutions. Most coaches are a combination of things.

In the past, I've hired two different types of personal trainers. The first one would say, "Come on! You can do one more!" The second one said, "Do you think you can do one more?" I learned that for me, the second type of coach is best. She made me want to try harder, to see if I could do just one more. The other one made me want to quit right then and say, "No! I can't!"

Decide which personality you need to support yours, and find that type of coach.

5. Look for a health coach with great troubleshooting skills.

It's one thing to work with your health coach when everything is going well. It's a whole different thing when you feel like you've done everything right, but the results you want keep slipping through your fingers.

This is where troubleshooting becomes really important. A fibromyalgia health coach with great troubleshooting skills will be able to discover what is blocking you, your health, and your progress. She can then help you get past those blocks, so you can start living the life you want to live.

When I managed a software support call center, I always instructed my staff, "Look for the question behind the question." This helps me today as a coach. Often the question you ask isn't the deeper question in your heart. There's usually a "question behind the question." For example, you might ask, "How can I stick to a gluten-free diet?" Or, "How can I make it easier to go to bed earlier?" Underneath it all, you might actually be thinking to yourself, "Why can't I take better care of myself? Why is this so hard?"

I could give you all kinds of advice on how to make better dietary choices or strategies for going to bed, but if we don't address the underlying questions, you'll just keep failing, over and over. You want a coach with killer troubleshooting skills.

6. *Choose how much time–and energy–you have to work on your health.*

Do you want a coach who can teach you how to grow, cook, and make everything from scratch; or, do you want a coach who will give you simple, practical ideas to make adding healthy habits into your life easier? Do you want to talk with your coach once a month? Or once a week?

I find with my clients that if it takes too much energy, or is too complicated, it just won't happen. As fibromyalgia patients, we have limited energy to begin with, am I right? If you somehow have the energy to go grocery shopping, then you don't have the energy to prepare a meal. If you have energy to prepare a meal, you don't have energy to clean up. And so on.

I also find that most health coaches want their clients to eat as close to natural as possible: clean, organic, homemade, and homegrown. I don't disagree with these concepts. I just understand that the real life of a fibromyalgia patient is something quite different.

What a fibromyalgia patient needs, and what most health coaches focus on, are often at odds with each other. This makes it even more important for you to interview potential coaches to make sure you're getting what you need.

Take a moment, as you're thinking about your search, to decide how much time you have to invest in changing your habits and your health–then find a coach who will provide you what you need for the time and energy you have.

7. Ask for a consultation to check for individualized coaching.

Fibromyalgia health coaching should be an individualized service. With something that varies as much as fibromyalgia symptoms do, a health coach should tailor their coaching to meet the specific needs of each client.

A consultation is a great way to find out if the health coach you're thinking about working with can offer you an individualized program. If you leave your consultation feeling like you received "cookie cutter" answers or a pre-printed solution, then keep looking!

8. Choose a coach with professional training and standards.

Not all coaches are equally qualified when it comes to having professional training or standards. As I discussed earlier, you want a coach who is a fibromyalgia expert–but you also want one who will protect your privacy, and keep up with the ethical standards of her profession.

As an indication of your coach's professionalism, you may want to look for her:

Contract. Most professional relationships include a contract. Why should coaching be any different? This contract would outline what you can expect from your health coach and what she expects from you. It will outline what you are receiving in coaching services, and what your coach is receiving in payment. If your coach is offering a guarantee, the contract should include it and outline what needs to happen in order for you to take advantage of it.

Willingness to stand behind her work. You've probably tried a lot of things that didn't work, and paid people who didn't always do what they promised. You want a coach who will stand behind her work.

Privacy policy. Health coaches that do not bill insurance aren't subject to HIPAA guidelines, like your doctor's office is. However, you still need to be confident that your personal information is safe and protected. After all, you'll be talking to your coach about your illness and other health concerns, not to mention potentially intimate details of your life.

Certification. This can provide you a certain level of confidence in your coach's skills. Anyone can call themselves a "coach." There's no industry standard for what a coach is. It's not like saying you're a doctor or a physical therapist. Looking for a Certified Health Coach will help you find someone who has been properly trained.

***

If you are interested in learning more about working with me, please visit my website: MyRestoredHealth.com. I invite you to schedule a consultation to see if we would be a good fit for each other. You can also sign up for my monthly email newsletter, or follow me on social media. I usually share tips on how to live well with fibromyalgia, current research, and stories of hope and encouragement.

CONCLUSION

Implementing a bunch of stuff all at once can be stressful–even if they're good, healthy things! Be kind to yourself and honor your body. Be gentle and go slow; start small. Choose the low hanging fruit. You can make the best use of the information in this book by beginning with one or two strategies that resonate the most. As you grow proficient at managing your fibromyalgia symptoms, you can always add new tools to your toolbox.

If you need any help deciding where to begin–or figuring out what will help you improve the most–please visit my website and schedule a consultation. I would love to help you take back your life!

ACKNOWLEDGEMENTS

Thank you to...

Fibromyalgia. Without you, I wouldn't have discovered my purpose in life. You have introduced me to some pretty extraordinary people and taught me so many lessons. I'm a better person and live an amazing life because of you.

All the doctors, patients, and advocates who have educated and inspired me along the way. For graciously answering my unending stream of medical questions, Dr. Kaley Bourgeois deserves extra thanks.

My clients: past, present, and future. It's quite possible that you have taught me more than I've taught you. This book is your book. I'm honored that you chose to share your journey with me.

My family. You helped me believe that I could be anything I wanted to be–and you didn't give me grief as I tried those different things on like clothes from Grama's dress-up trunk. And thanks, Mom, for reading this *just one more time.*

My husband. You are my knight in black leather, on a horse with two wheels. Every girl should be rescued as often and as well as you have rescued me. You have saved the day AGAIN! You are my rock and my best friend. I love you.

The Great Storyteller. You chose to write my life as a redemption story and use my pain to help others. For that, I will always be grateful.

ABOUT THE AUTHOR

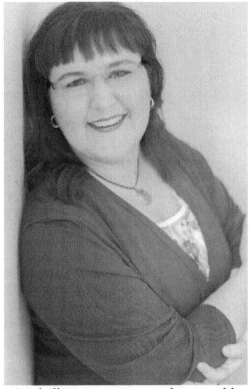

Tami Stackelhouse encourages hope and healing as a coach, author, speaker, and patient advocate. A fibromyalgia patient herself, Tami has gone from disabled to thriving. Her compassion, gentle support, and fun coaching style help women with fibromyalgia take back control of their lives.

Healthline named Tami's blog as one of the 15 Best Fibromyalgia Blogs of 2015 for its quality and contribution to the fibromyalgia community. Tami is a Certified Health Coach and has been a panelist and presenter for organizations such as the Oregon Fibromyalgia Information Foundation and Molly's Fund Fighting Lupus. She is a graduate of the Leaders Against Pain Scholarship Training sponsored by the National Fibromyalgia & Chronic Pain Association (NFMCPA), and a member of the Leaders Against Pain Action Network.

As a patient advocate, Tami began working with the NFMCPA and Oregon doctors in 2013 to petition policymakers to move fibromyalgia onto the Prioritized List of conditions covered by Medicaid reimbursement. As of 2015, that battle is still ongoing. In 2015, Tami coordinated efforts that resulted in Governor Kate Brown signing a proclamation honoring May 12th as Fibromyalgia Awareness Day for the state of Oregon.

Tami lives in the suburbs of Portland, with her husband, Scott, and their three cats: Sam, Jesse, and Sniglets. On sunny days, you'll find her on the back of Scott's Harley. When it's raining, she will be by the fire, reading a good book, and rubbing Sam's Belly of Happiness and Joy.

Connect with Tami online at:
Website and blog: MyRestoredHealth.com
Facebook: www.facebook.com/FibroCoach
Twitter: www.twitter.com/FibroCoach
Pinterest: www.pinterest.com/FibroCoach

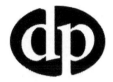

ABOUT DIFFERENCE PRESS

Difference Press offers life coaches, other healing professionals, a comprehensive solution to get their book written, published, and promoted. A boutique style alternative to self-publishing, Difference Press boasts a fair and easy to understand profit structure, low priced author copies, and author-friendly contract terms. Founder, Angela Lauria has been bringing the literary ventures of authors-in-transformation to life since 1994.

Your Delicious Book

If you're like many of the authors we work with, you have wanted to write a book for a long time, maybe you have even started a book … or two… or three … but somehow, as hard as you have tried to make your book a priority other things keep getting in the way.

It's not just finding the time and confidence to write that is an obstacle. The logistics of finding an editor, hiring an experienced designer, and figuring out all the technicalities of publishing stops many authors-in-transformation from writing a book that makes a difference. Your Delicious Book is designed to address every obstacle along the way so all you have to do is write!

Tackling The Technical End Of Publishing

The comprehensive coaching, editing, design, publishing and marketing services offered by Difference Press mean that your book will be edited by a pro, designed by an experienced graphic artist, and published digitally and in print by publishing industry experts. We handle all of the technical aspects of your book creation so you can spend more of your time focusing on your business.

Ready To Write Your Book?

Visit www.YourDeliciousBook.com. When you apply mention you are Difference Press reader and get 10% off the program price.

OTHER BOOKS BY DIFFERENCE PRESS

Scale: Refuse to Settle, Recognize What Matters, Redefine Success
by Travis Collier

The Mother Within: A Guide To Accepting Your Childless Journey
by Christine Erickson

It's Not Rocket Science: Leading, Motivating and Inspiring Your Team To Be Their Best
by Susan Foster

Every Time I Diet I Gain 5 Pounds: Step Into Your True Self And Shed Your Baggage
by Galina Knopman

ClutterFree Revolution: Simplify Your Stuff, Organize Your Life & Save The World
by Evan Michael Zislis

Vibe Your Way to Fit, Healthy, & Hot
by Charity Gonzalez

Money Mindset for a Champagne Life
by Cassie Parks

Three Guys Walk into a Bar: How To Thrive As A Creative Business
by Jim Shields

SPECIAL OFFER

Congratulations!
By reading this book, you have taken a great step towards taking back your life. I want to take a moment here to honor that. Remember what I said earlier: "90% of the medical care you receive comes from YOU." Kudos for picking up this book and reading it!

At the same time, how much you improve, and how good you feel, is directly related to the actions and attitude you have towards yourself. This means that the real work of getting well depends on where you go from here. Simply reading this book isn't enough. You need to incorporate the ideas and information into your life for things to change.

I've created several worksheets and videos to help you do just that. These resources are usually only available to my coaching clients and workshop attendees. However, I am making them available as my gift to you. I know they will make it easier for you to implement these ideas and *Take Back Your Life*. Download these bonus items at: MyRestoredHealth.com/book-bonuses.

It was impossible for this book to contain everything I know about how to live a great life with fibromyalgia. I'm definitely going to be writing more. In the meantime, I invite you to schedule a consultation with me, at no charge, to discuss your unique set of symptoms and challenges. I know what it's like to feel like a prisoner in your own body. I would love to help you *Take Back Your Life.*

[1]Savastio, Rebecca. "Fibromyalgia Mystery Finally Solved!" *Guardian Liberty Voice*. 20 Jun 2013. Web. 20 Apr 2015. <http://guardianlv.com/2013/06/fibromyalgia-mystery-finally-solved/>.

[2]Richards, Karen Lee. "History of Fibromyalgia." *Health Central*. 16 Mar 2009. Web. 11 May 2015. <http://www.healthcentral.com/chronic-pain/fibromyalgia-287647-5.html>

[3]Inanici, F. Yunus MB. "History of Fibromyalgia: Past to Present." *Curr Pain Headache Rep*. 2004 Oct;8(5):369-78. Web. 11 May 2015. <http://www.ncbi.nlm.nih.gov/pubmed/15361321>

[4]University Of Michigan Health System. "Fibromyalgia Pain Isn't All In Patients' Heads, New Brain Study Finds." ScienceDaily. 7 June 2002. <www.sciencedaily.com/releases/2002/06/020607073056.htm>.

[5]Rice, Frank L. "Women with Fibromyalgia Have A Real Pathology Among Nerve Endings to Blood Vessels in the Skin." Integrated Tissue Dynamics. 24 Jun 2013. Web. 20 Apr 2015. <http://www.intidyn.com/images/pdfs/Fibromyalgia_Pathology_for_lay_people_2013-06-24.pdf>

[6]Rice, Frank L. "Fibromyalgia Is Not All In Your Head, New Research Confirms." Integrated Tissue Dynamics. 14 Jun 2013. Web. 20 Apr 2015.
<http://www.intidyn.com/news-events/news/20-researchers-discover-a-rational-biological-source-of-pain-in-the-skin-of-patients-with-fibromyalgia-press-relase>

[7]Jesús Castro-Marrero, Mario D. Cordero, Naia Sáez-Francas, Conxita Jimenez-Gutierrez, Francisco J. Aguilar-Montilla, Luisa Aliste, and José Alegre-Martin. Antioxidants & Redox Signaling. November 20, 2013, 19(15): 1855-1860. doi:10.1089/ars.2013.5346. Web. 21 Apr 2015.
<http://online.liebertpub.com/doi/abs/10.1089/ars.2013.5346>

[8]Sánchez-Domínguez, Benito, et al. "Oxidative stress, mitochondrial dysfunction and, inflammation common events in skin of patients with Fibromyalgia." *Mitochondrion* 21 (2015): 69-75.
<http://www.sciencedirect.com/science/article/pii/S1567724915000215>

[9]Katz, Robert S., and Anthony Farkasch. "The Straight Neck in Fibromyalgia." *Arthritis and Rheumatism.* Vol. 65. 111 River Street, Hoboken, NJ 07030-5774, USA: Wiley-Blackwell, 2013. Web. 21 Apr 2015.
<http://www.fmcpaware.org/fibromyalgia/research-abstracts/1478-the-straight-neck-in-fibromyalgia-abstract.html>

[10]Savvas Radević. Tender points fibromyalgia svg.svg. Creative Commons license:
<http://commons.wikimedia.org/wiki/File:Tender_points _fibromyalgia_svg.svg>

[11]Hultquist, Pattie Brynn. "Confessions of a Superhero..." *Lupus Interrupted.* 29 May 2011. Web. 23 Apr 2015. <http://www.lupusinterrupted.com/confessions-of-a-superhero/>

[12]Harker KT, Klein RM, Dick B, Verrier MJ, Rashiq S. "Exploring attentional disruption in fibromyalgia using the attentional blink." Psychol Health. 2011 Jul;26(7):915-29. doi: 10.1080/08870446.2010.525639. Epub 2011 Jun 1. Web. 19 Apr 2015. <http://www.ncbi.nlm.nih.gov/pubmed/21598187>

[13]American College of Rheumatology, 2010. <https://www.rheumatology.org/Practice/Clinical/Patient s/Diseases_And_Conditions/Fibromyalgia/>

[14]Bennett, Robert M et al. "An Internet Survey of 2,596 People with Fibromyalgia." *BMC Musculoskeletal Disorders* 8 (2007): 27. PMC. Web. 16 Apr. 2015. <http://www.ncbi.nlm.nih.gov/pmc/articles/PMC1829161/>

[15]Anson, Pat. "New Fibromyalgia Blood Test is 99% Accurate." *National Pain Report.* 30 Jul 2013. Web. 19 Apr 2015.

<http://nationalpainreport.com/new-fibromyalgia-blood-test-is-99-accurate-8821072.html>

[16]Anson, Pat. "New Fibromyalgia Blood Test is 99% Accurate." *National Pain Report.* 30 Jul 2013. Web. 19 Apr 2015.
<http://nationalpainreport.com/new-fibromyalgia-blood-test-is-99-accurate-8821072.html>

[17]Anson, Pat. "Fibromyalgia Blood Test Gets Insurance Coverage." Pain News Network. 27 May 2015. Web. 22 Jun 2015.
<http://www.painnewsnetwork.org/stories/2015/5/27/fibr omyalgia-blood-test-gets-insurance-coverage>

[18]Bennett, Robert M., et al. "An internet survey of 2,596 people with fibromyalgia." *BMC musculoskeletal disorders* 8.1 (2007): 27. Web. 22 Apr 2015.
<http://www.biomedcentral.com/1471-2474/8/27#>

[19]Bennett, Robert M. "OHSU/NFMCPA Survey of Symptoms Other than Pain for FDA Meeting Part 1." National Fibromyalgia & Chronic Pain Association. Web. 22 Apr 2015 <http://www.fmcpaware.org/ohsu-nfmcpa-survey-of-symptoms-other-than-pain-for-fda-meeting-part-1.html>

[20]Bennett, Robert M. "OHSU/NFMCPA Survey of Symptoms Other than Pain for FDA Meeting Part 2." National Fibromyalgia & Chronic Pain Association. Web. 22 Apr 2015. <http://www.fmcpaware.org/ohsu-nfmcpa-

survey-of-symptoms-other-than-pain-for-fda-meeting-part-2.html>

[21]Sarzi-Puttini P., et al. "Fibromyalgia syndrome: the pharmacological treatment options." Reumatismo. 2008 Jul-Sep;60 Suppl 1:50-8. Web. 4 May 2015. <http://www.ncbi.nlm.nih.gov/pubmed/18852908>

[22]Cunningham, M. O., Woodhall, G. L., Thompson, S. E., Dooley, D. J. and Jones, R. S. G. (2004), Dual effects of gabapentin and pregabalin on glutamate release at rat entorhinal synapses *in vitro*. *European Journal of Neuroscience*, 20: 1566–1576. doi: 10.1111/j.1460-9568.2004.03625.x. Web. 11 May 2015. <http://onlinelibrary.wiley.com/doi/10.1111/j.1460-9568.2004.03625.x/abstract>

[23]Harris, R. E., Sundgren, P. C., Craig, A. D., Kirshenbaum, E., Sen, A., Napadow, V. and Clauw, D. J. (2009), Elevated insular glutamate in fibromyalgia is associated with experimental pain. *Arthritis & Rheumatism,* 60: 3146–3152. doi: 10.1002/art.24849. Web. 11 May 2015. <http://onlinelibrary.wiley.com/doi/10.1002/art.24849/abstract>

[24]Younger, Jarred, Luke Parkitny, and David McLain. "The Use of Low-Dose Naltrexone (LDN) as a Novel Anti-Inflammatory Treatment for Chronic Pain." *Clinical Rheumatology* 33.4 (2014): 451–459. *PMC*. Web. 10 May 2015. <http://www.ncbi.nlm.nih.gov/pmc/articles/PMC3962576/>

[25]Younger, J., Noor, N., McCue, R. and Mackey, S. (2013), Low-dose naltrexone for the treatment of fibromyalgia: Findings of a small, randomized, double-blind, placebo-controlled, counterbalanced, crossover trial assessing daily pain levels. Arthritis & Rheumatism, 65: 529–538. Web. 3 May 2015.
<http://www.ncbi.nlm.nih.gov/pubmed/23359310>
University Of Michigan Health System. "Fibromyalgia Pain Isn't All In Patients' Heads, New Brain Study Finds." ScienceDaily. 7 June 2002.
<www.sciencedaily.com/releases/2002/06/020607073056.htm>.

[27]Itoh K, Kitakoji H. Effects of acupuncture to treat fibromyalgia: A preliminary randomised controlled trial. *Chinese Medicine*. 2010;5:11. doi:10.1186/1749-8546-5-11. Web. 3 May 2015.
<http://www.ncbi.nlm.nih.gov/pmc/articles/PMC2852376/>

[28]University of Michigan Health System. "Chinese acupuncture affects brain's ability to regulate pain, study shows." 10 Aug 2009. Web. 3 May 2015. <http://www.uofmhealth.org/news/1246chinese-acupuncture-effects>

[29]Okie S. A Flood of Opioids, a Rising Tide of Deaths. *The New England Journal of Medicine.* 18 Nov 2010. Web. 3 May 2015.
<http://www.nejm.org/doi/full/10.1056/NEJMp1011512>

[30]Consumer Pain Advocacy Task Force. "What We Believe." Web. 3 May 2015.
<http://consumerpainadvocacy.org>

[31]Castro-Marrero J, et al. "Could mitochondrial dysfunction be a differentiating marker between chronic fatigue syndrome and fibromyalgia?" Antioxid Redox Signal. 2013 Nov 20;19(15): 1855-60. doi: 10.1089/ars.2013.5346. Epub 2013 May 29. PubMed PMID: 23600892. Web. 28 Jun 2014.
<http://www.ncbi.nlm.nih.gov/pubmed/23600892>

[32]Jacob E. Teitelbaum, Clarence Johnson, and John St. Cyr. "The Use of D-Ribose in Chronic Fatigue Syndrome and Fibromyalgia: A Pilot Study." The Journal of Alternative and Complementary Medicine. November 2006, 12(9): 857-862. doi:10.1089/acm.2006.12.857. Web. 5 May 2015.
<http://online.liebertpub.com/doi/abs/10.1089/acm.2006. 12.857>

[33]Costantini A, et al. "High-dose thiamine improves the symptoms of fibromyalgia." BMJ Case Rep. 2013 May 20;2013. pii: bcr2013009019. doi: 10.1136/bcr-2013-009019. PubMed PMID: 23696141. Web. 28 Jun 2014.
<http://www.ncbi.nlm.nih.gov/pubmed/23696141>

[34]O'Brien, Sharon M. Detecting sleep abnormalities early helps reduce fibromyalgia risk. Clinical Advisor. 6 Apr 2012. Web. 9 Apr 2015.

<http://www.clinicaladvisor.com/detecting-sleep-abnormalities-early-helps-reduce-fibromyalgia-risk/printarticle/235479/>

[35]Liptan, Ginevra (2011-01-31). Figuring out Fibromyalgia: Current Science and the Most Effective Treatments (Kindle Locations 447-449). Visceral Books. Kindle Edition.

[36]Blue light has a dark side. Harvard Health Publications. 1 May 2012. Web. 11 Apr 2015.
<http://www.health.harvard.edu/staying-healthy/blue-light-has-a-dark-side>

[37]Srinivasan, V., Lauterbach, E. C., Ho, K. Y., Acuña-Castroviejo, D., Zakaria, R., & Brzezinski, A. (2012). Melatonin in Antinociception: Its Therapeutic Applications. Current Neuropharmacology, 10(2), 167–178. doi:10.2174/157015912800604489
<http://www.ncbi.nlm.nih.gov/pmc/articles/PMC3386506/>

[38]Wilhelmsen, M., Amirian, I., Reiter, R. J., Rosenberg, J. and Gögenur, I. (2011), Analgesic effects of melatonin: a review of current evidence from experimental and clinical studies. Journal of Pineal Research, 51: 270–277. doi: 10.1111/j.1600-079X.2011.00895.x
<http://onlinelibrary.wiley.com/doi/10.1111/j.1600-079X.2011.00895.x/abstract>

[39]Wikner, J., Hirsch, U., Wetterberg, L. and Röjdmark, S. (1998), Fibromyalgia — a syndrome associated with

decreased nocturnal melatonin secretion. Clinical Endocrinology, 49: 179–183. doi: 10.1046/j.1365-2265.1998.00503.x
<http://onlinelibrary.wiley.com/doi/10.1046/j.1365-2265.1998.00503.x/abstract>

[40]Blue light has a dark side. Harvard Health Publications. 1 May 2012. Web. 11 Apr 2015.
<http://www.health.harvard.edu/staying-healthy/blue-light-has-a-dark-side>

[41]Herman, John. Ultimate Light Bulb Test: Incandescent vs. Compact Fluorescent vs. LED. Popular Mechanics. Web. 11 Apr 2015.
<http://www.popularmechanics.com/technology/gadgets/reviews/g164/incandescent-vs-compact-fluorescent-vs-led-ultimate-light-bulb-test/>

[42]"sleep hygiene". Oxford Dictionaries. Web. 11 Apr 2015.
<http://www.oxforddictionaries.com/us/definition/american_english/sleep-hygiene>

[43]Foerster, B. R., Petrou, M., Edden, R. A. E., Sundgren, P. C., Schmidt-Wilcke, T., Lowe, S. E., … Harris, R. E. (2012). Reduced Insular γ-Aminobutyric Acid in Fibromyalgia. *Arthritis and Rheumatism*, *64*(2), 579–583. doi:10.1002/art.33339
<http://www.ncbi.nlm.nih.gov/pmc/articles/PMC3374930/>

[44]Sun ER, Chen CA, Ho G, Earley CJ, Allen RP. Iron and the restless legs syndrome. *Sleep.* 1998 Jun 15;21(4):371-7. <http://www.ncbi.nlm.nih.gov/pubmed/?term=9646381>

[45]Monsein M, Corbin TP, Culliton PD, Merz D, Schuck EA. Short-term outcomes of chronic back pain patients on an airbed vs innerspring mattresses. *MedGenMed.* 2000 Sep 11;2(3):E36. <http://www.ncbi.nlm.nih.gov/pubmed/11104482>

[46]http://www.cdc.gov/nchs/data/ahcd/namcs_summary/2010_namcs_web_tables.pdf

[47]Rabin, Roni Caryn. 15-Minute Visits Take A Toll On The Doctor-Patient Relationship. *Kaiser Health News.* 21 Apr 2014. Web. 10 Apr 2015. <http://kaiserhealthnews.org/news/15-minute-doctor-visits/>

[48]"advocate." Easton's 1897 Bible Dictionary. 15 Apr. 2015. <Dictionary.com http://dictionary.reference.com/browse/advocate>.

[49]"self-care." The American Heritage® Stedman's Medical Dictionary. Houghton Mifflin Company. 18 Jan. 2015. <Dictionary.com http://dictionary.reference.com/browse/self-care>.

[50]Miserandino, Christine. "The Spoon Theory." ButYouDontLookSick.com. 2010. 7 Apr 2015.

<http://www.butyoudontlooksick.com/articles/written-by-christine/the-spoon-theory/>

[51]Brooks, Havi. "*The Book of You*." The Fluent Self. 30 Mar 2010. 5 Apr 2015.
<www.fluentself.com/blog/stuckification/the-book-of-you/>

[52]AAFP.org, Health coaching dramatically lowers patients' systolic blood pressure, 4 Jul 2012.
http://annfammed.org/content/10/3/199.full.pdf+html

[53]Thom, David H. et al. "The impact of health coaching on medication adherence in patients with poorly controlled diabetes, hypertension, and/or hyperlipidemia: a randomized controlled trial." Journal of the American Board of Family Medicine January-February 2015 vol. 28 no. 1 38-45. PMC. Web. 3 Apr. 2015.
http://www.jabfm.org/content/28/1/38.long

[54]Leahey, Tricia M., and Rena R. Wing. "A Randomized Controlled Pilot Study Testing Three Types of Health Coaches for Obesity Treatment: Professional, Peer, and Mentor." Obesity (Silver Spring, Md.) 21.5 (2013): 10.1002/oby.20271. PMC. Web. 3 Apr. 2015.
http://www.ncbi.nlm.nih.gov/pmc/articles/PMC3484232/

[55]Adams SR, Goler NC, Sanna RS, Boccio M, Bellamy DJ, Brown SD, et al. Patient Satisfaction and Perceived Success with a Telephonic Health Coaching Program: The Natural Experiments for Translation in Diabetes (NEXT-D) Study, Northern California, 2011. Prev Chronic Dis

2013;10:130116.   DOI:
http://dx.doi.org/10.5888/pcd10.130116
http://www.cdc.gov/pcd/issues/2013/13_0116.htm